RADIOLOGY FOR BEGINNERS

A Journey Inside the Human Body

SOPHIA AISHWARYA LI

ISBN:

First Edition

Printed in the USA

ACKNOWLEDGMENTS

Many thanks to all the radiologists and trainees who encouraged and supported me whilst writing this book. It wouldn't have been possible without you. Special thanks to Dr. Peter Julien, Chief of Chest Imaging Radiology, who fact-checked and helped to make this a credible source of information for teenagers, pre-med, and medical students looking for inspiration in regard to a future career.

For my grandmother,
who loves me unconditionally
and has never stopped believing in me.

CONTENTS

CHAPTER 1

INTRODUCTION TO THE WORLD OF RADIOLOGY

Would you like to sneak a peek inside the human body and solve puzzles all day long for a career? Does examining parts of the human body, using beautiful pictures that are almost unimaginable and have been captured by amazing, cutting-edge technology, sound appealing? One of the primary responsibilities of a radiologist is acting as a detective, figuring out if a crime of the organs has been committed and the patient should be detained in hospital or if the body is acquitted and the person is free to go home. A radiologist is not what one typically thinks of as a doctor; they are not like your usual pediatrician or surgeon. Radiologists are medical doctors who examine pictures taken inside the patient to determine the cause of the patient's symptoms. They do not take the pictures themselves, however. There are cameramen behind the scenes to take pictures for them, called radiology technologists (techs), who specialize in the different types of pictures taken, such as X-rays, ultrasound, computed tomography scans (CTs) and magnetic resonance imaging (MRI).

In this book, we are going to explore the images of the body that can be obtained from a CT scan, as it is the easiest to understand, and its principles can be applied to other imaging modalities. The radiologist's job is to act as the translator or interpreter of the images produced by the CT scanner or through MRIs, X-rays, or ultrasounds. Some sub-specialties of radiology involve performing procedures that don't involve cutting the body open. With the use of imaging techniques, the radiologist can guide the needle into the correct part of the body and take samples for biopsy; insert a drain; or even give treatment to a tumor, so the patient does not have to undergo an extensive surgery. Isn't it cool to be able to look inside the human body without having to cut it open? This book will contain some fascinating images of certain parts of the body, both normal and abnormal, so you can also practice being a detective of disease.

CHAPTER 2

WHAT LIES BENEATH: EXPLORING THE ABDOMEN

Now it is time to dive deep into the mysterious world of the abdomen. What do you think of when you hear the word "belly"? It is home to our favorite snacks, occasional food babies, and a whole bunch of important organs.

When it comes to exploring the abdomen with radiology, things can get pretty interesting. Just imagine peeking inside your own body, without having to perform any surgery—now that's what we call modern magic! With the help of CT scans, MRIs and ultrasounds, we can see everything from your stomach to your intestines, all without making a single incision. It's like a high-tech game of hide-and-seek, but with organs instead of toys.

But wait—there's more! Not only can we explore the abdomen with radiology, but we can also spot any pesky disease that might be lurking. From appendicitis to gallstones, our trusty CT scans can help us catch these troublemakers before they cause too much mischief.

Now, before you start panicking about all the potential issues hiding in your abdomen, remember that knowledge is power. By understanding the anatomy of your belly and how radiology can help us to see what's going on inside, you'll be better equipped to take care of your body. Plus, who knows? You might even discover a newfound appreciation for those organs that work tirelessly to keep you up and running.

Let's get started by learning how to first start looking at CT scans. You know what they say: a picture is worth a thousand words.

ABDOMINAL IMAGING

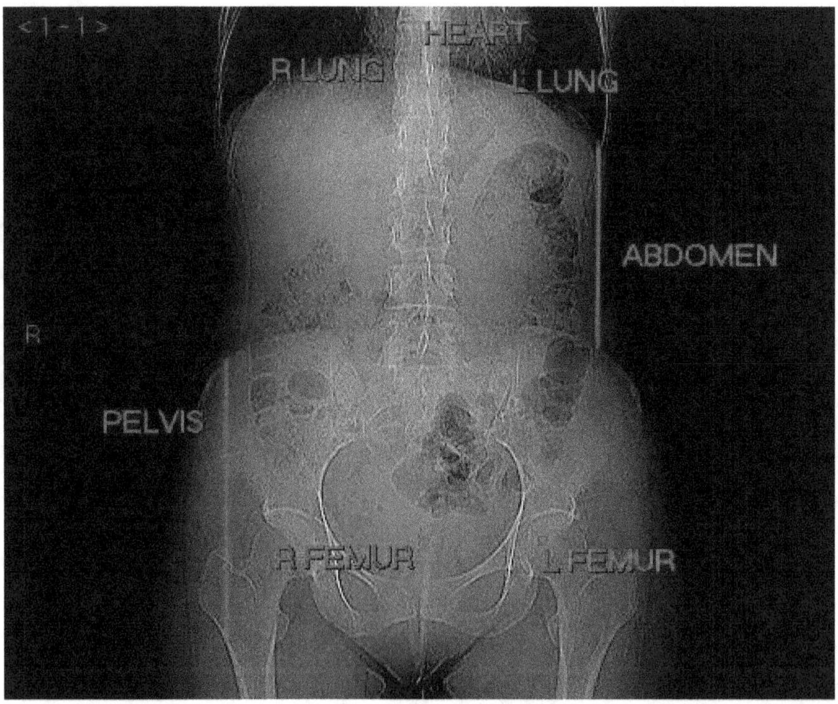

Figure 1. A frontal CT scout view (topogram) of the abdomen.

First, the area to be scanned must be determined, which is done by the CT scout view (topogram), based on what part of the human body the doctor has ordered to be scanned. In the case of the abdomen and pelvis, this CT scout view (*Figure 1*) demonstrates that the scan begins at the lung bases and covers the abdomen and pelvis, extending to below the top of the femurs, the thigh bones, and the hip bones, which is the standard. This topogram is similar in appearance to an X-ray of the abdomen.

The way that CT scans are read or interpreted is as if we are slicing through the patient's body, similarly to a slice of cake, from the head to the feet, which is called the **axial** view. The right-hand side of the body as depicted on the CT scan is a person's left-hand side, and the CT's scan left-hand perspective is a person's right-hand side. This may seem confusing at first, but just think about the CT scan being inverted, like one of those filters on TikTok which flips your face the other way around.

The abdomen may be a mysterious place, but, with the power of radiology on our side, we can unravel its secrets and keep our bodies in tip-top shape. We will now be taking a dive into what is normal and abnormal by looking at one organ at a time. It is important to understand normal anatomy to be able to distinguish what is malignant and a disease from something that is harmless and benign.

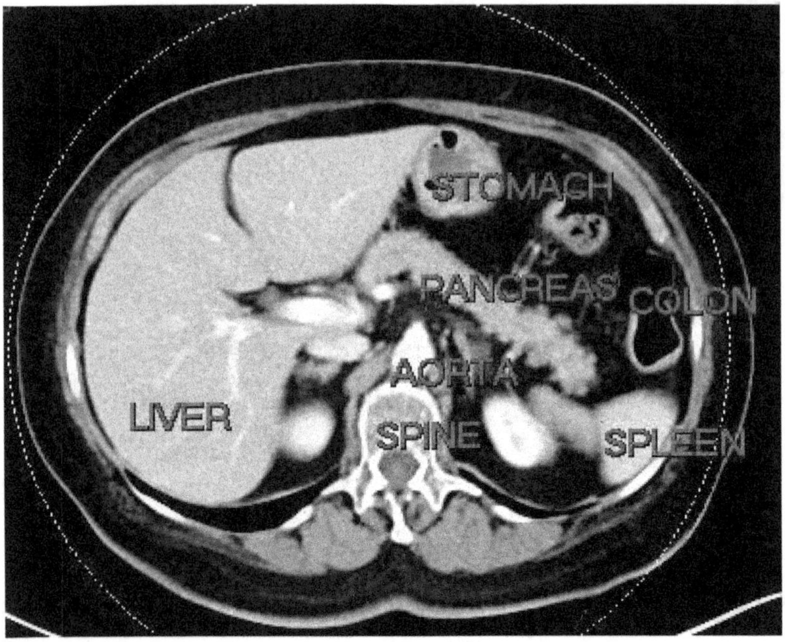

Figure 2.An axial image (slice) through the mid abdomen.

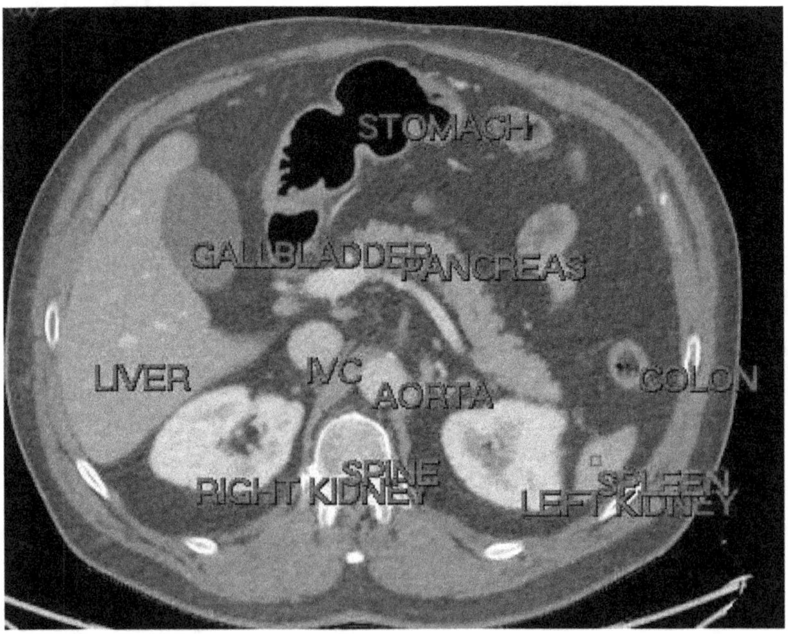

Figure 3.An axial image through the mid abdomen slightly lower than in Figure 2.

First, we will be covering the normal anatomy of the body. In *Figures 2* and *3*, the organs are clearly labeled. The stomach is the organ at the top of the scan, with the black coloring displaying the gas inside. The gallbladder is pictured in a darker grey and is positioned next to the liver, pictured in a lighter grey, on the right side of the body. The pancreas, which looks like a feather, is positioned near the gallbladder. The inferior vena cava (IVC), the biggest vein in the body, is represented as a white dot that lies slightly to the right of the aorta (the biggest artery in the body). Additionally, there are two kidneys on either side of the spine; a spleen, which is in the left upper abdomen; and a colon, which looks a little like a picture frame because it wraps around the small intestine. It is difficult to identify the colon wrapping around in this particular image (Figure 3), because the image shown represents only a slice of the body taken from top to bottom. However, from a coronal view (as depicted in Figure 4) it is easier to see, because the scanner would be slicing from front to back, as if you are looking at the front of the body. If these terms seem unfamiliar, you are in luck! This book will describe the function and importance of each organ and vein spoken about above.

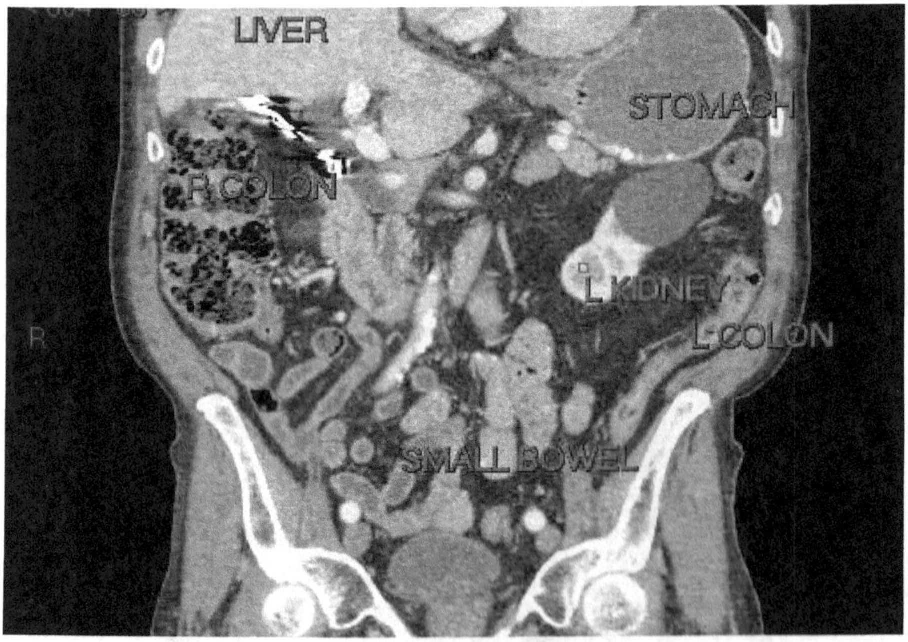

Figure 4. A coronal image through the mid abdomen.

This first coronal image (*Figure 4*) shows the small bowel in the center. The large bowel, labelled as R colon (right colon), and L colon (left colon) are to the left- and right-hand sides of the picture frame consecutively.

As we scan more towards the front of the abdomen, the transverse colon, which is the longest part of the large intestine, comes into view in the horizontal upper frame. See *Figure 5*.

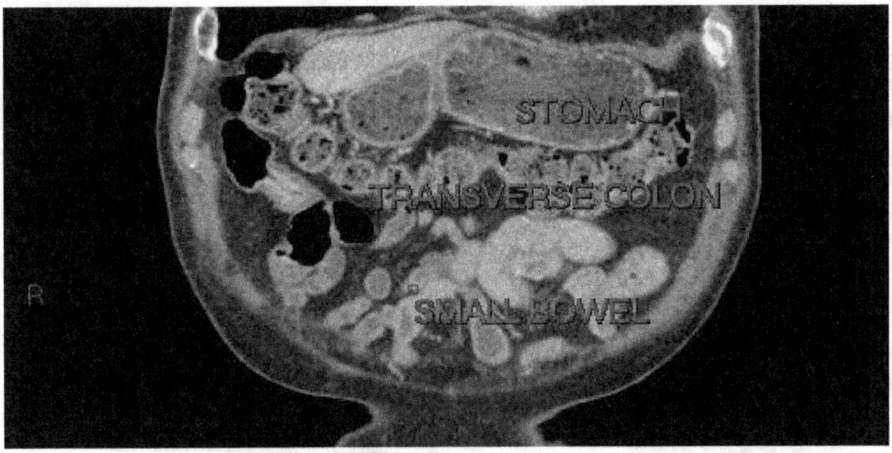

Figure 5. A coronal image through the mid abdomen slightly more anterior or towards the front.

Now we have a little bit of the lay of the land, let's dive a little deeper into the normal organs, what they look like, where they live, and what their purpose is in keeping our bodies alive and healthy.

THE LIVER

Let's start with the biggest organ of a normal abdomen: the **liver**. The liver is a large main organ located in the right side of the body, which filters all the blood; breaks down poisonous substances, such as drugs and alcohol; produces bile to help break down fats, digest food and remove waste; regulates blood clotting; and assists in resisting infections. It is said the liver is similar in size to a football. The average size of the liver is between 13- 16cm for the right lobe measured vertically. A liver that is larger than 17cm is considered large. If you were to view the liver in real life, it would be a dark reddish-brown and normally shaped like a cone or wedge. On a CT scan, the organs are different shades of grey.

BENIGN LIVER ABNORMALITIES

The most common type of lesion in the liver is a cyst. The **liver cyst** is the homogenous grey structure in the left liver, circled in *Figure 6.* Nearly all liver cysts are benign (noncancerous) and are fluid-filled sacs that usually don't grow large enough to cause symptoms.

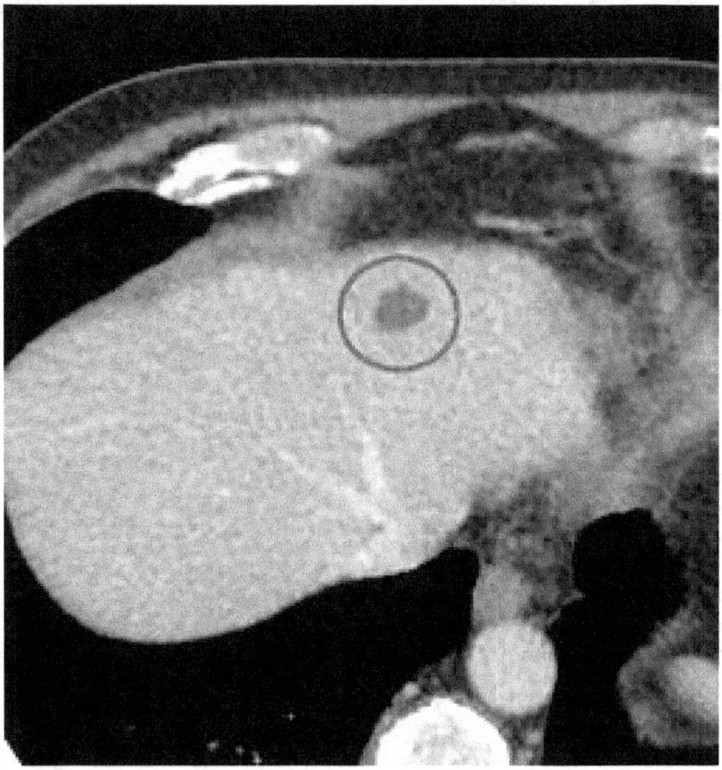

Figure 6. Circled is a small hepatic cyst.

The next most common liver lesion or spot is called a **hemangioma**, which has a classic type of look, called peripheral nodular enhancement, meaning there are little dots of nodules in the periphery, resembling a string of pearls in a pearl necklace (*Figure 7*). This can be diagnosed on a CT as a benign entity made up of a tangle of vessels. Hemangiomas also rarely require treatment, except for when they are over 10cm.

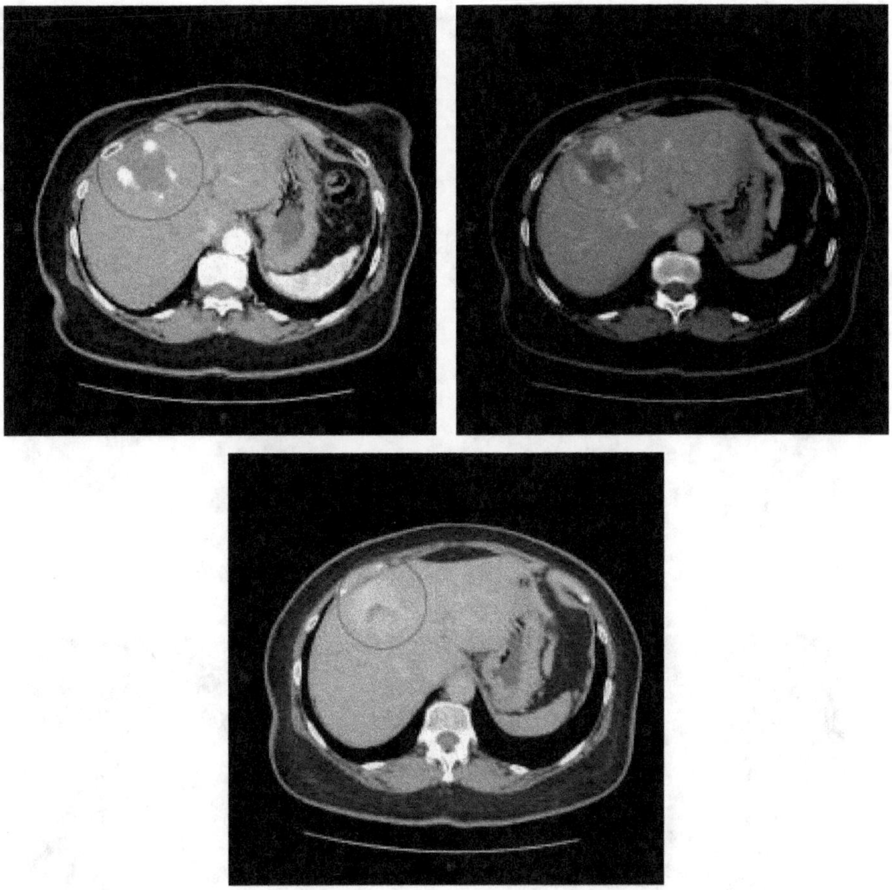

Figure 7. The liver lesion circled above demonstrates progressive nodular peripheral contrast filling with increased slow filling from the first arterial phase to the second venous phase and then the last delayed image that is classic for a hemangioma.

MALIGNANT LIVER ABNORMALITIES

We now turn to masses that are malignant. The origin of the cancer is called the primary; when the mass spreads to a different organ, the site of its spread is called a **metastasis**. *Figure 8* shows one liver metastasis, which is circled; *Figure 9* shows multiple enlarging masses that are liver metastases. These are cancerous tumors that have spread to the liver from other parts of the body. This is bad news.

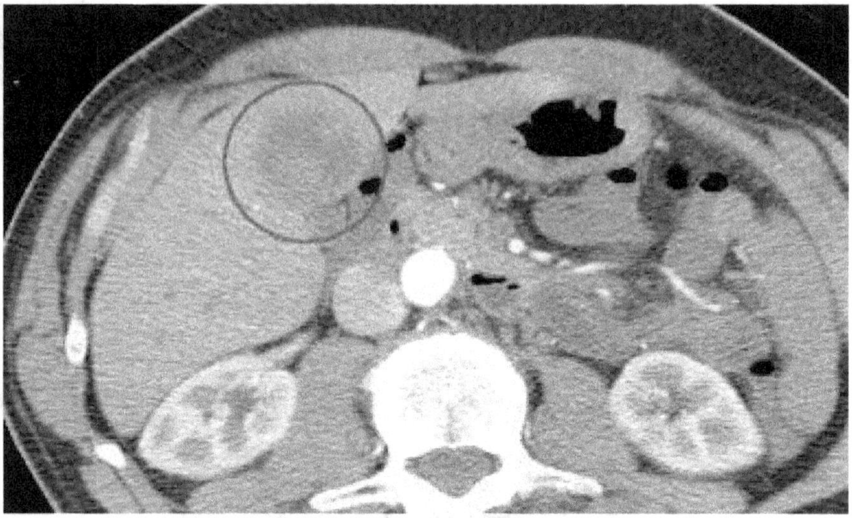

Figure 8. An axial CT image with a liver metastasis contained in the circle.

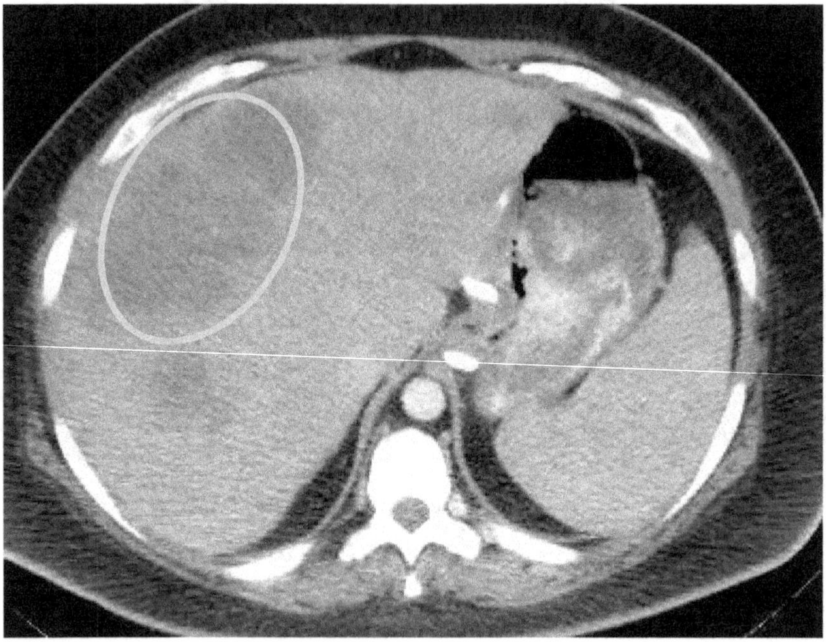

Figure 9. Enlarging hepatic(relating to the liver) metastases.

Sometimes, the whole liver is affected by a disease. **Cirrhosis** is scarring of the liver caused by long-term liver damage. During later stages, one may experience yellowing of the skin or jaundice. With cirrhotic liver, the liver shrivels up, usually as a result of too much regular alcohol consumption or a condition such as hepatitis, which can be caused by intravenous drug use. As you can see, when compared to the liver in *Figure 6*, this liver pictured in *Figure 10* has an irregular surface when it should be smooth.

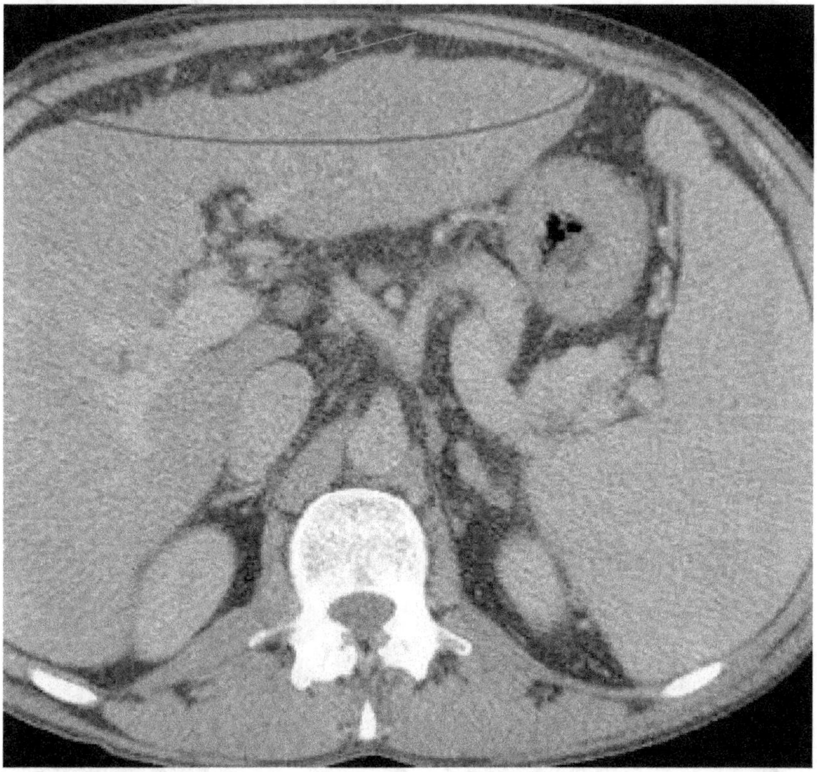

Figure 10.A CT scan demonstrating the nodular surface of a cirrhotic liver.

THE ADRENAL GLANDS

The **adrenal glands**, also known as suprarenal glands, are located at the top of both kidneys. Adrenal glands are the fight-or-flight organs. Their function is to produce hormones that help to regulate your metabolism, immune system, blood pressure and response to stress. In terms of appearance, they are V-shaped or triangular in appearance and approximately 2–5cm in size.

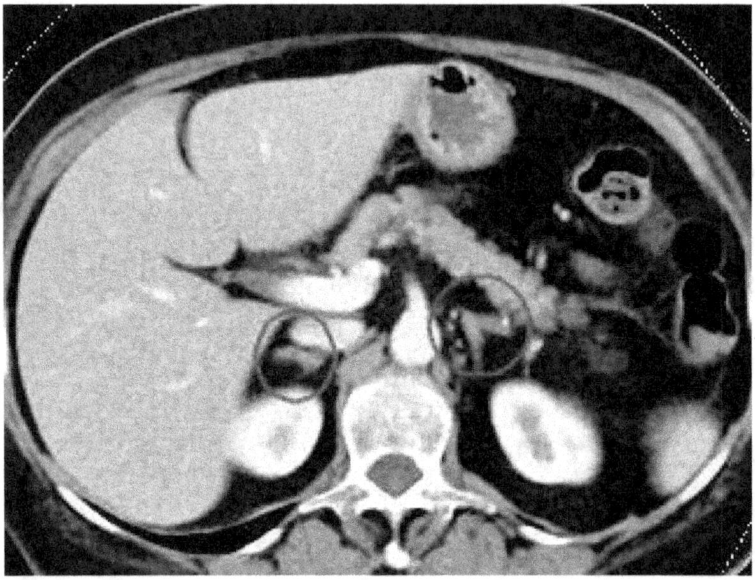

Figure 11.Circled are the paired adrenal glands which have an inverted V shape.

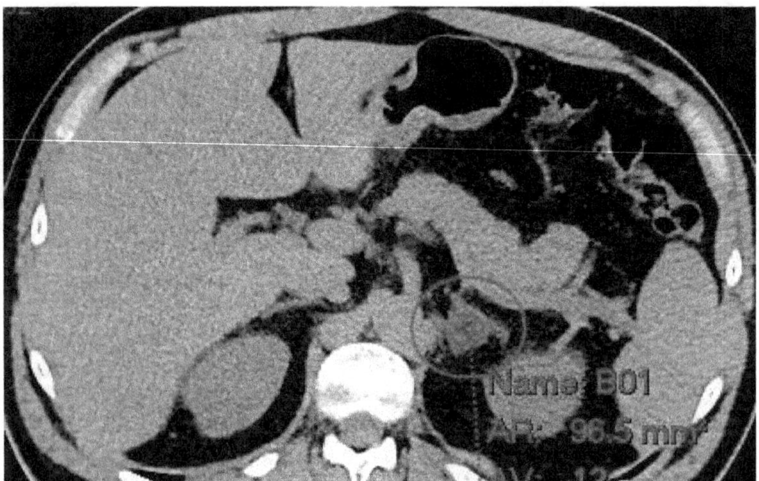

Figure 12.Circled is an enlarged rounded left adrenal with low density below 10 Hounsfield Units representing an adenoma.

ADRENAL ABNORMALITIES

When an adrenal abnormality becomes overactive, it can become a round nodule called an **adenoma**, instead of its normal V-shape. To ensure it's a benign adenoma, radiologists' pair a measuring structure with the CT scan to calculate the density. If it is below 10 Hounsfield units on a non-contrast CT (no dye), it is a benign adenoma. Contrast is dye that makes everything light up. A Hounsfield unit is also known as a CT unit, which is a relative quantitative measurement of radio density. You don't need to know exactly what it is, but just be aware that radiologists use Hounsfield units to measure the density of something and determine whether it is fat, fluid, or bone. *Figure 12* displays a benign adenoma, which is under 10 Hounsfield units and is circled. All adenomas are benign. If something is over 10 Hounsfield units, it could be a cancer or metastatic (spread from a cancer), rather than an adenoma.

THE KIDNEYS

Next on the list to investigate at the crime scene are the kidneys. There are two **kidneys**, which are located just below the ribcage and on either side of the spine. The kidneys filter blood and regulate a balance of water, salts, and minerals in the body. Every minute, the kidneys filter about a half a cup of blood, removing extra water and waste to produce urine. They are bean-shaped, each about the size of a fist.

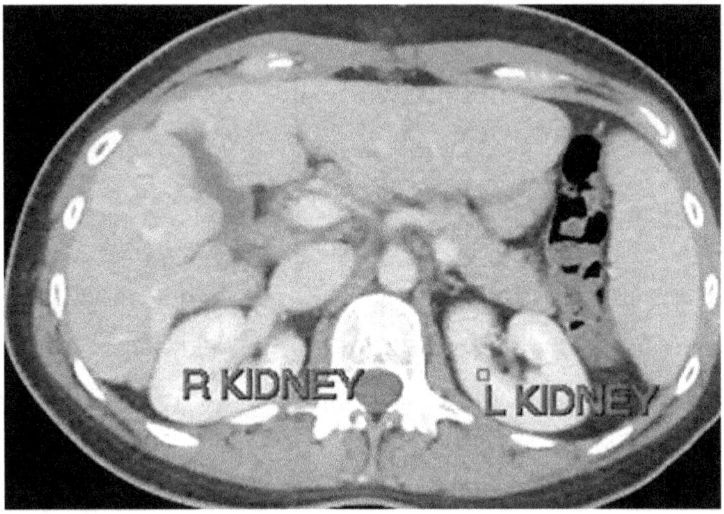

Figure 13. Labelled are the right and left kidney on either side of the spine.

KIDNEY ABNORMALITIES

A CT scan can assess whether a mass in the kidney is benign or otherwise. To ascertain whether a mass enhances/has vascularity (blood flow) and could be malignant, the technologist injects a dye through the veins, which reaches all the organs and lights them up.

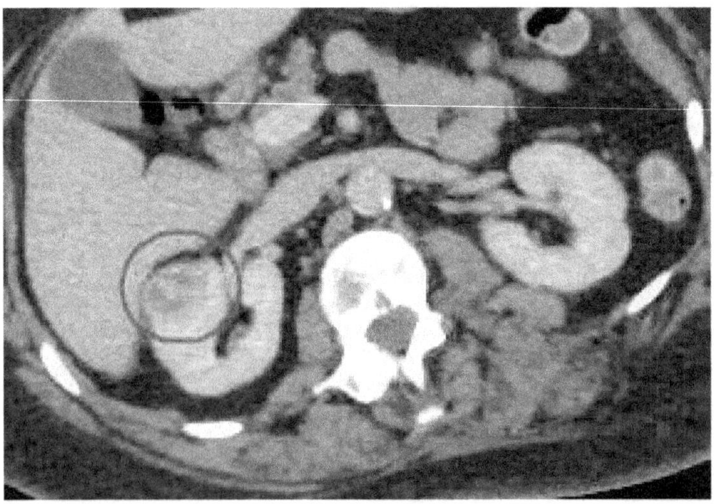

Figure 14. Circled is a mixed enhancing right kidney mass.

Figure 14 is an example of a CT with contrast given. When a kidney mass enhances—meaning that it lights up after contrast (dye) is given—(and doesn't contain fat which is black on a CT scan), this is likely to be a **renal** (related to the kidneys) **cancer**, until proven otherwise. It's important to catch these early, so that it does not have the opportunity to become larger or metastasize. About 50% of renal cancers are incidentally detected by imaging such as CTs, ultrasounds and MRIs performed for other purposes, so imaging can really save lives. In *Figure 14*, you can see the difference between the left and right kidney; the kidney with renal cancer is circled. It has enlarged, becoming a large blob. If untreated, it can resemble the kidney presented in *Figure 15*, which depicts renal cancer that has taken over the entire right kidney.

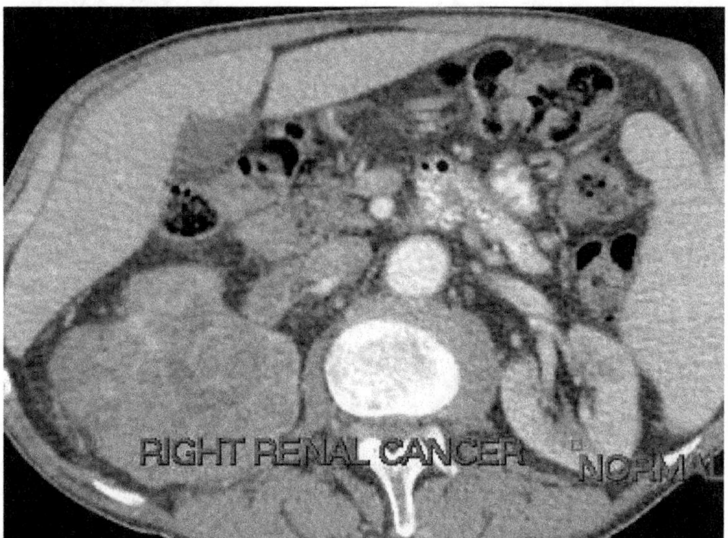

Figure 15.The right kidney is replaced by a large mass.

One thing to look for is fat within the renal mass. Fat shows up as black on a CT scan, which you can see surrounding the abdomen beneath the skin in *Figure 15*. When a renal mass contains fat, it is called an **angiomyolipoma** and signifies that it is benign.

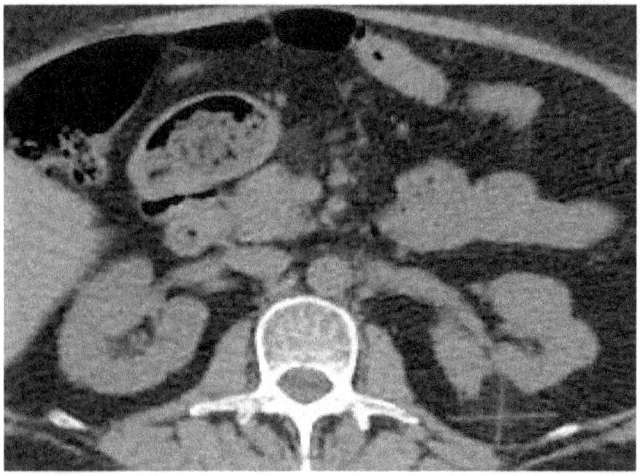

Figure 16.The cross hairs measure a fat density mass that blends in with the fat that surrounds the left kidney and so can be characterized as an angiomyolipoma.

In *Figure 16*, the left kidney has an angiomyolipoma. Angiomyolipomas are benign, so they can be left alone; however, when they become large or over 4cm, there is potential for bleeding in the kidney. If they do bleed, an interventional radiologist can embolize (a procedure that uses particles, such as tiny gelatin sponges or beads, to block a blood vessel) the artery in question, stopping blood flow without a huge surgery.

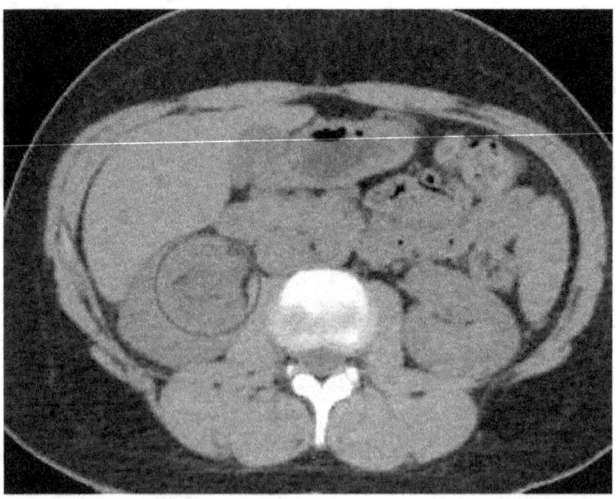

Figure 17.Noncontrast axial CT image with the right kidney collecting system circled, where urine travels from the kidney to the bladder. Note that this is more full and bulbous compared to the normal left kidney collecting system.

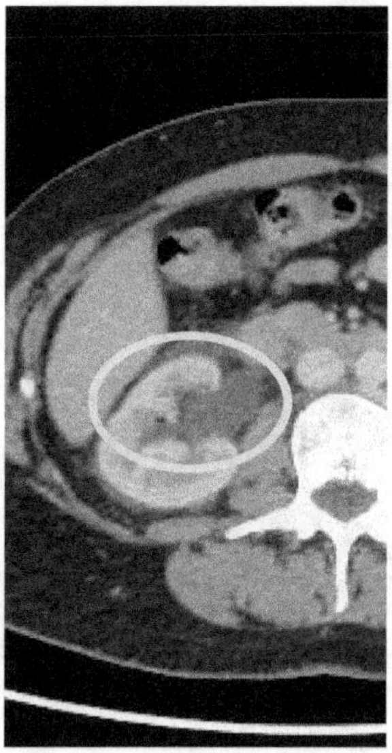

Figure 18.The fullness of the right renal collecting system is circled representing mild right hydronephrosis. This is better seen when contrast is given which enhances the right kidney cortex – the urine does not enhance.

When the kidney gets blocked, this is called **<u>hydronephrosis</u>**, which can cause excruciating pain. *Figure 17* is without contrast (dye), so everything is pictured in different shades of grey; an enlargement of the drainage system for the right kidney is circled. This is better seen when contrast is given (*Figure 18*); in this image, depicted in white and grey, it can be seen that the kidney lights up. Hydronephrosis can cause swelling of one or both kidneys due to a buildup of urine. In *Figures 17* and *18*, the right kidney outflow pipe is blocked, so it has become enlarged. With a CT scan, one can also often find the cause of the blockage.

Stones from the blocked kidneys can pass down the pipe that extends from the kidney to the bladder, called the ureters, which can cause hydronephrosis. These stones block the kidney and can cause it to stop functioning. When the stones are small (typically less than 5mm), they can pass into the bladder and then can be urinated out; however, when they are larger, a surgeon may have to intervene. *Figure 19* depicts a tiny ureterovesical junction stone, - that means at the junction between the ureter (the pipe draining the urine) and the bladder (the organ that stores urine, with "vesical" meaning relating to the bladder) as the cause for the hydronephrosis. A stone of this size can be left to pass on its own.

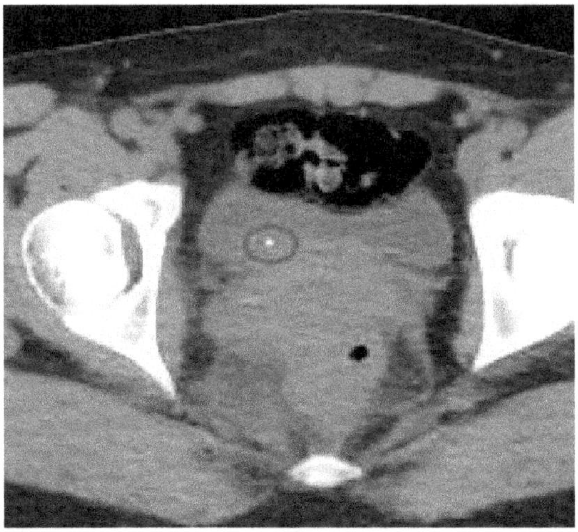

Figure 19. A tiny calcification lies at the junction between the right ureter and bladder.

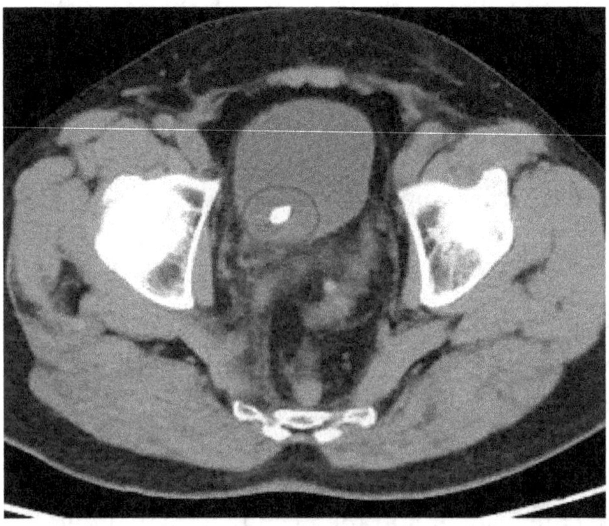

Figure 20. A larger stone lies in a similar location to that of Figure 19.

It is difficult to know if the stone has already passed into the bladder (in which case it will just be expelled when the person goes to the bathroom) or whether it is still within the junction and requires surgery. What can be helpful is turning the patient upside down to perform the CT scan.

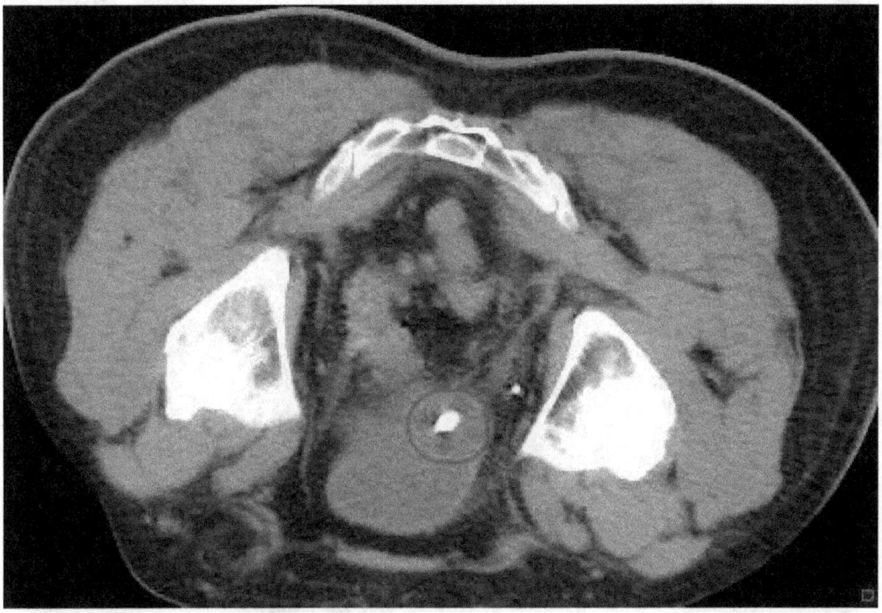

Figure 21.Prone imaging- when the patient lies on their stomach -helps tell whether the stone is at the junction between the ureter and bladder or has passed into the bladder.

Figure 21 shows that when the patient is put upside down, the stone does not fall to the bottom of the bladder, so therefore it can not be passed out with the next "number 1". The stone is still located at the ureterovesical junction, so a surgeon specializing in kidneys (the urologist) can treat this to improve the patient's kidney function.

THE SPLEEN

The **spleen** is located opposite the liver in the left upper abdomen. It is a small organ whose job is to fight off infections and control the level of blood cells. The spleen is soft and dark purple, and is shaped like a very small catcher's mitt, with notches on its upper front. The weight and size of the spleen can vary, but the average healthy adult's spleen is less than 12cm in length and about 6 ounces in weight.

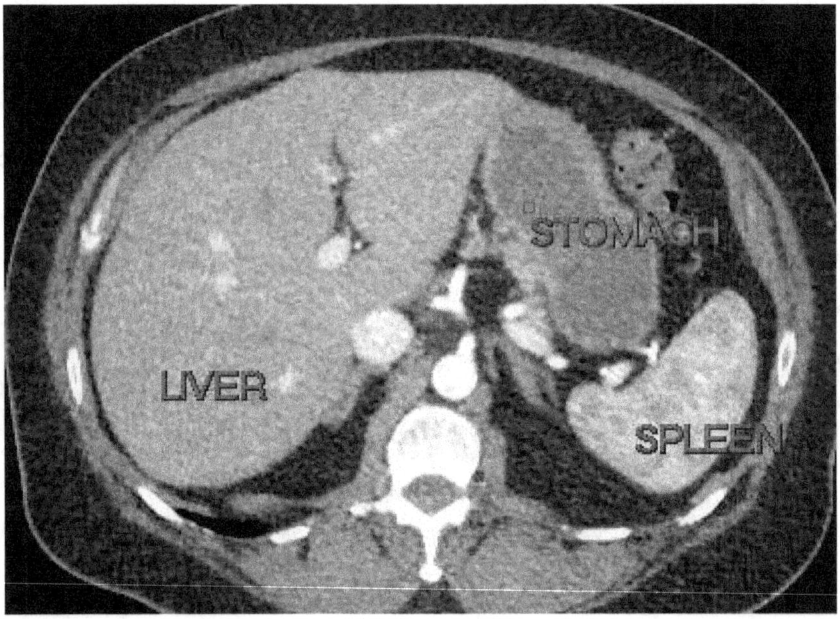

Figure 22.Labelled are the spleen in the left upper abdomen, the liver in the right upper abdomen and the stomach containing liquid.

ABNORMALITIES OF THE SPLEEN.

As the normal spleen is less than 12cm in length, a diameter of 13cm usually indicates enlargement, which is called **splenomegaly**. There are several reasons that the spleen can become enlarged. Some common reasons are viral infections, such as mononucleosis ("mono", also known as the kissing disease); cirrhosis; and blood cancers, such as leukemia and lymphoma.

The spleen can become injured; there are different grades of injury. Circled in *Figure 22* on the left of the body is a **ruptured spleen**, with blood surrounding it. If an injury to the spleen is too extensive, it must sometimes be removed.

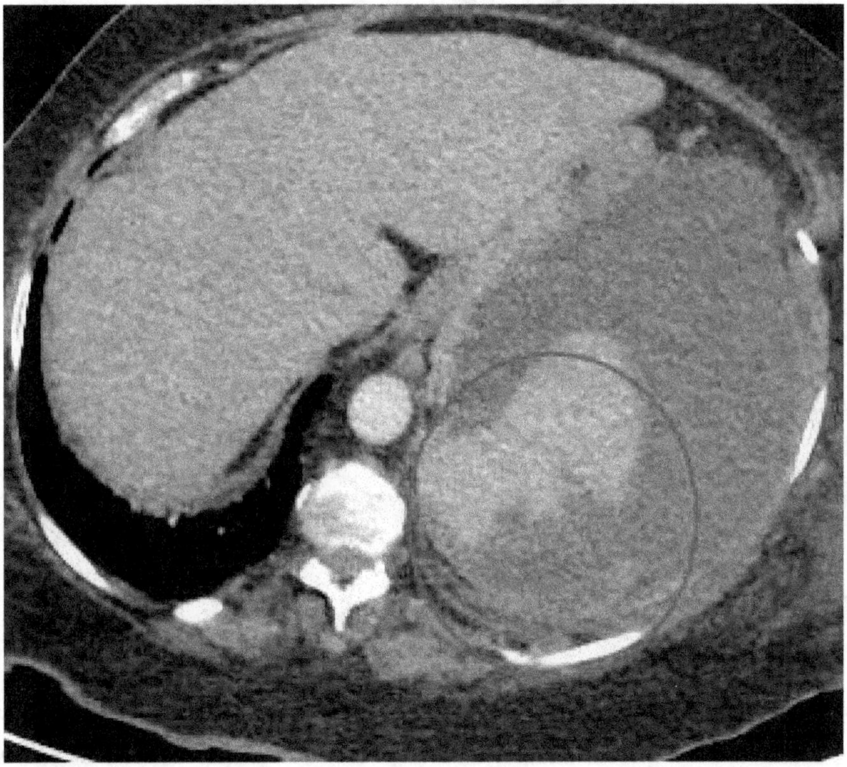

Figure 22.Circled is the area where the spleen has ripped apart- called a splenic rupture.

When a part of an organ dies, it is called an **infarct**. *Figure 23* shows an infarct of the spleen; in other words, part of the spleen has died. The darker grey that is circled is the infarct.

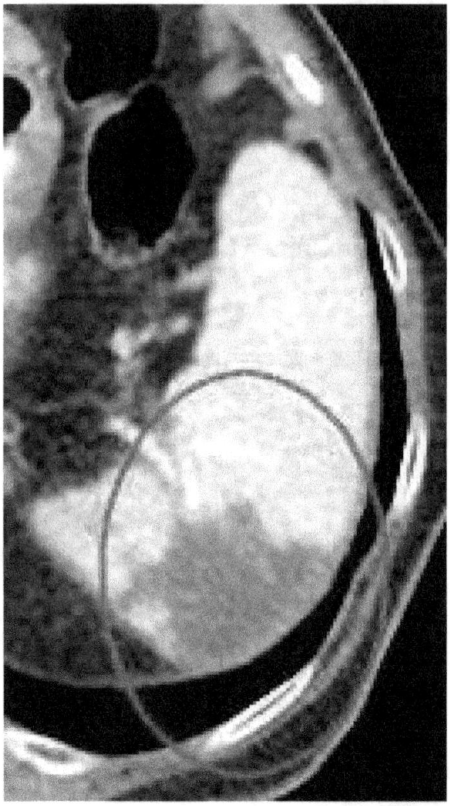

Figure 23. Circled is an area of lack of enhancement within the otherwise enhancing spleen and this represents a portion of dead spleen called an infarct.

THE PANCREAS

In between the liver and spleen, in the middle of the body, is the **pancreas**. The pancreas performs two main functions: an exocrine function, in which the pancreas releases enzymes, such as protein, to aid digestion; and an endocrine function, which produces insulin, a hormone that aids in controlling blood sugar levels. The pancreas is a sausage-shaped structure with a fluffy, feathery appearance. It is about 15cm (6 inches) in length.

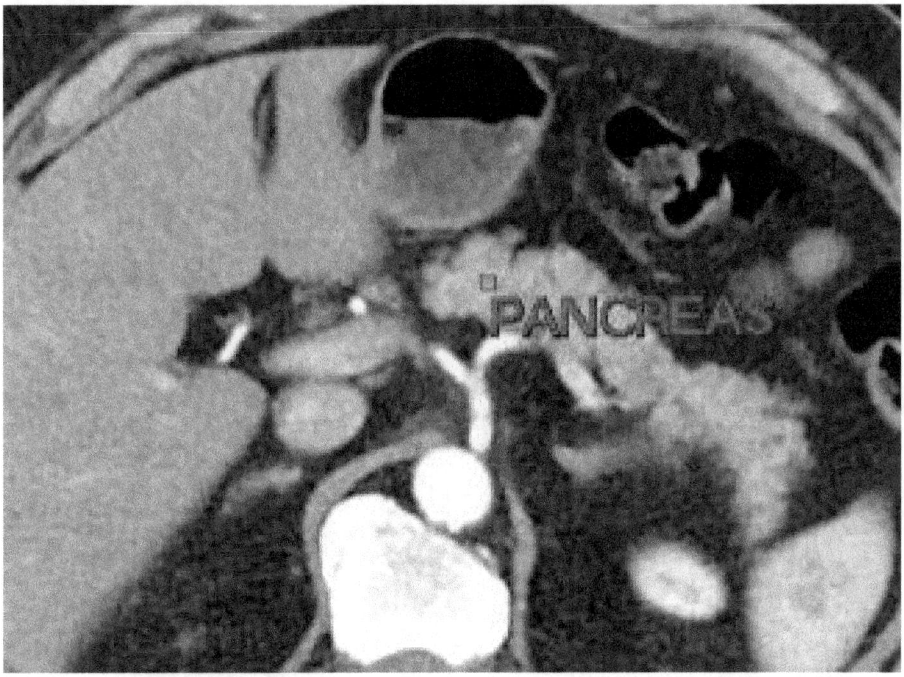

Figure 24. The fluffy organ in the center of the abdomen is labelled as the pancreas.

PANCREATIC ABNORMALITIES

Figure 24 depicts a normal pancreas. When the pancreas becomes angry and inflamed, this is called **pancreatitis**. "Itis" means inflammation, so when anything becomes inflamed, an "itis" is added on the end. The most common causes of pancreatitis are gallstones and overconsumption of alcohol. When pancreatitis occurs, the pancreas looks fuzzy and swollen, because it has been surrounded by fluids, and lacks its normal feathery appearance (*Figure 25*). If you are feeling severe stomach pain that may spread to your back or chest, nausea, vomiting, or a rapid heart rate, you may be experiencing pancreatitis. These are symptoms shared with many abnormalities, so don't worry—you may just have a common cold.

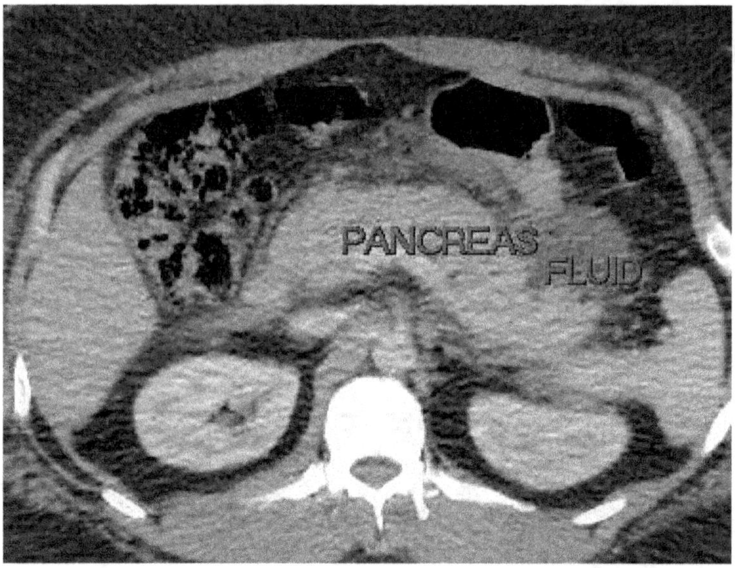

Figure 25. The pancreas is shown to be swollen, ill defined and with surrounding fat stranding suggesting inflammation. The grey area that is not enhancing next to the pancreas is fluid which can also develop as a complication of pancreatitis, sometimes becoming loculated.

THE GALLBLADDER

The **gallbladder** is a fluid-filled structure that lies in the right upper abdomen, next to the liver. It stores and releases bile, which is fluid that helps to digest fats. The gallbladder is a wide, pear-shaped sac in appearance, measuring around 4cm wide and 7–10cm long.

GALLBLADDER ABNORMALITIES

The formation of gallstones happens when bile stored in the gallbladder hardens to stone-like material. Gallstones are like marbles that can cause pain in your right upper abdomen. Gallstones can sometimes be seen, and there are several ways gallstones can appear. As on the CT scan in *Figure 26*, there are two gallstones, highlighted by an arrow. These are depicted in black on the CT scan, as they are made of nitric oxide. Sometimes, gallstones can also appear as little calcified balls lying within the gallbladder, as circled in *Figure 27*.

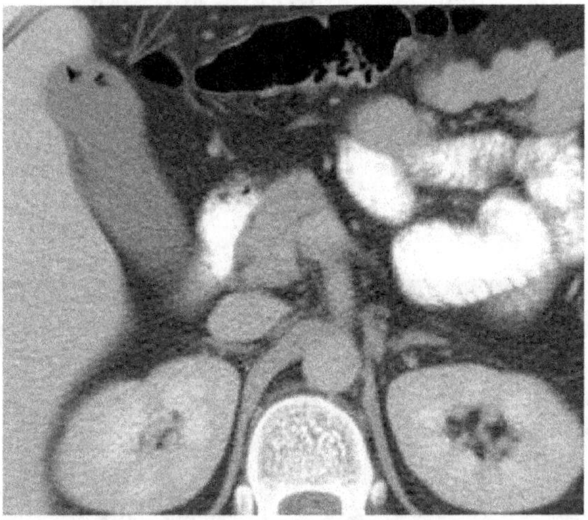

Figure 26. The arrow points to two gallstones. These have the Mercedes- Benz sign which is gas (nitric oxide)within the stones causing this typical appearance.

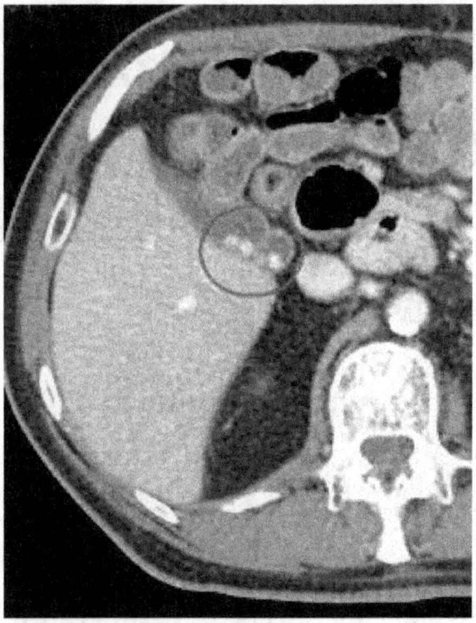

Figure 27. The dependent white marble like structures that are circled are calcified gallstones falling into the gallbladder.

If gallstones are not visible on a CT scan, this does not mean they are not present, as CT is not as good at picking them up as some other imaging methods, such as ultrasound and MRI. CT is useful for identifying kidney stones, picking up 99% of them, but those in the gallbladder can still be missed when it comes to a CT scan. Ultrasound is better at finding gallstones, which look like marbles in a bag, as circled in *Figure 28.*

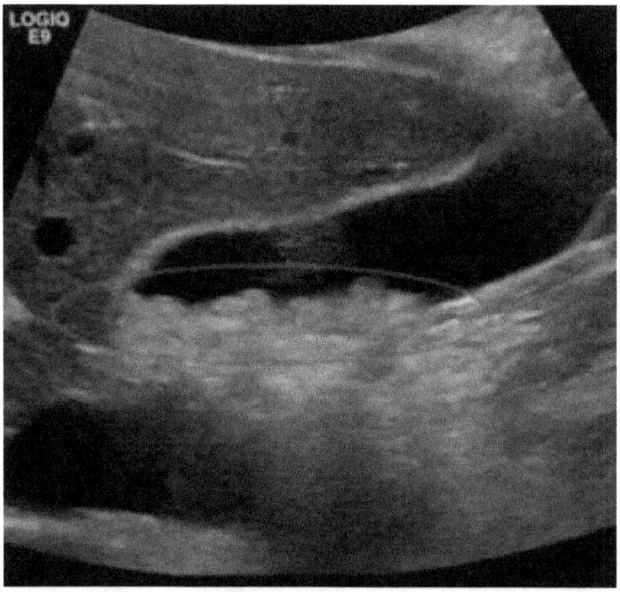

Figure 28. Ultrasound images showing marble like structures layering in the gallbladder with shadows behind them representing gallstones.

Another good way of detecting gallstones is MRI. MRI images are created when patients lie in an MRI scanner (a large, tube-shaped magnet), which uses a combination of radio waves and a strong magnetic field to produce detailed images of the inside of the body. We cannot delve into all the wonderful aspects of MRI in this book, but we can get a glimpse of how the abdomen can look and the crispness of the images obtained by MRI. As you can see, from being aware of where all the

organs live in the abdomen through CT, we can then locate and get detailed pictures of any abnormalities on MRI.

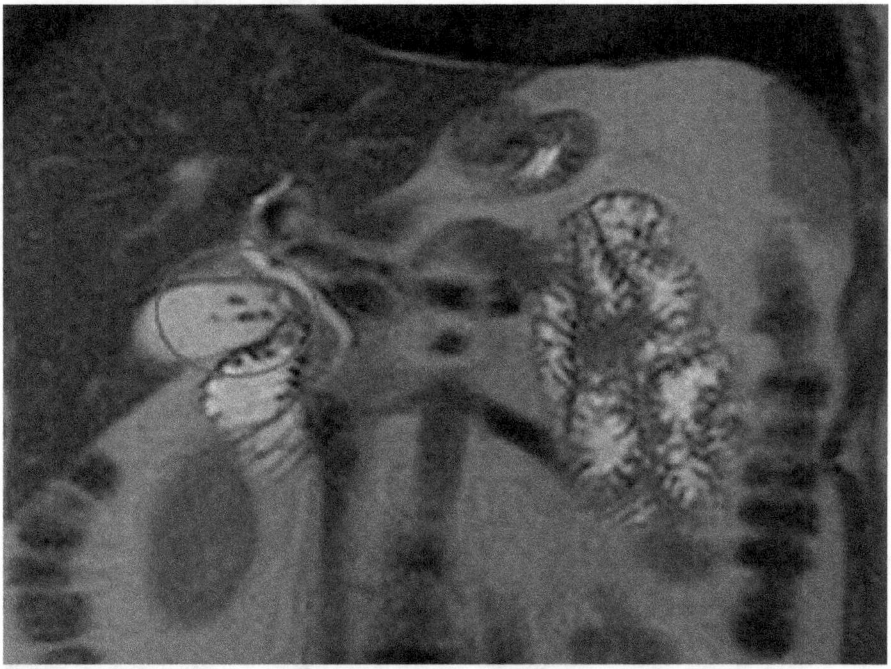

Figure 29. A coronal MRI image showing the gallbladder as a fluid filled structure (white on this sequence) with tiny balls which represent gallstones.

As seen in the MRI image in *Figure 29*, slicing through the abdomen from front to back (coronal images), the white blob that is circled is the gallbladder containing fluid, with the marbles located inside being the gallstones.

THE APPENDIX

So, what exactly is the **appendix**? It's a small, finger-shaped pouch, located at the beginning of your large intestine. It's not exactly the most glamorous organ in your body, but it does serve a purpose (or it used to). Scientists believe that the appendix may have once been used to help digest tough plant materials, but nowadays it's pretty much useless.

THE SCOOP ON APPENDICITIS

Let's talk about **appendicitis**—the classic "my stomach hurts" diagnosis. This pesky little organ called the appendix can cause a whole lot of trouble when it becomes inflamed. However, fear not, because CT scans are here to save the day, by helping doctors to pinpoint the exact location of the problem and decide whether surgery is necessary. Just remember—if you're experiencing sharp pain in your lower right abdomen, it might be time to pay a visit to the radiology department.

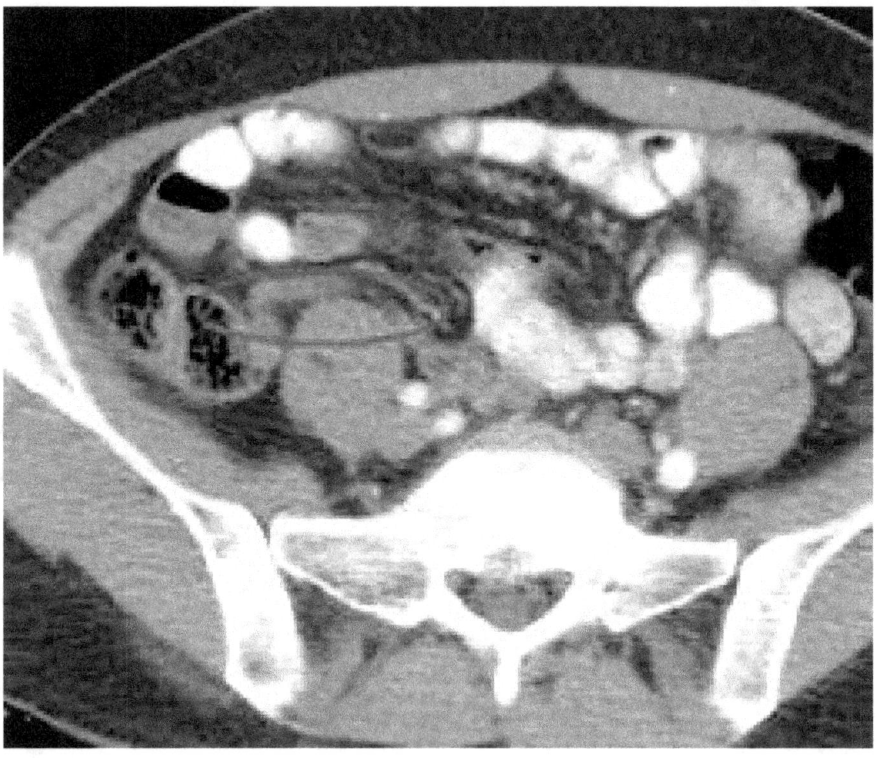

Figure 30. Axial CT image showing the normal appendix circled.

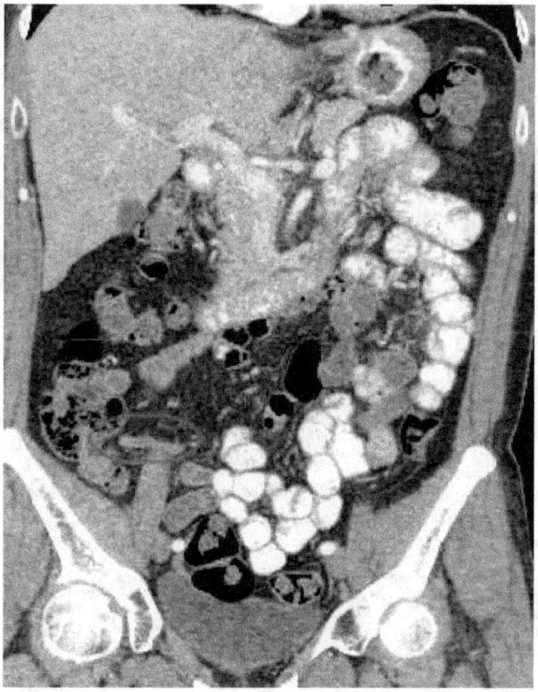

Figure 31. Coronal CT image showing the normal appendix circled.

The normal appendix is less than 6mm in width and looks like the little tube circled on the axial image in *Figure 30* and on the coronal image in *Figure 31*. It is located in the right lower abdomen at the base of the colon. If that seems difficult to find, just remember the appendix is connected to the bottom of the cecum, otherwise known as the base of the right large intestine. That might make your detective work a little easier.

In *Figure 32*, you can see how thick and inflamed the appendix has become— it is definitely larger than 6mm—which indicates appendicitis. A diagnosis of appendicitis is dependent on size, so if the appendix seems large and inflamed, it is certainly a warning sign. Now the surgeon is aware, the appendix should be removed to make the patient feel better.

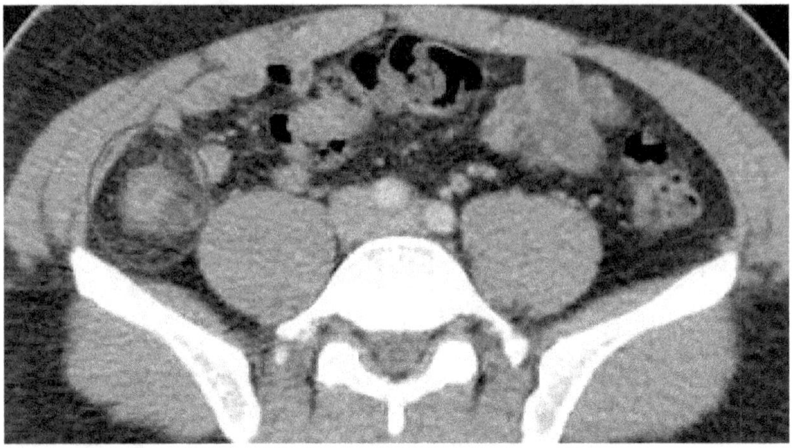

Figure 32. Fat stranding and enlargement of the appendix implies inflammation and therefore appendicitis.

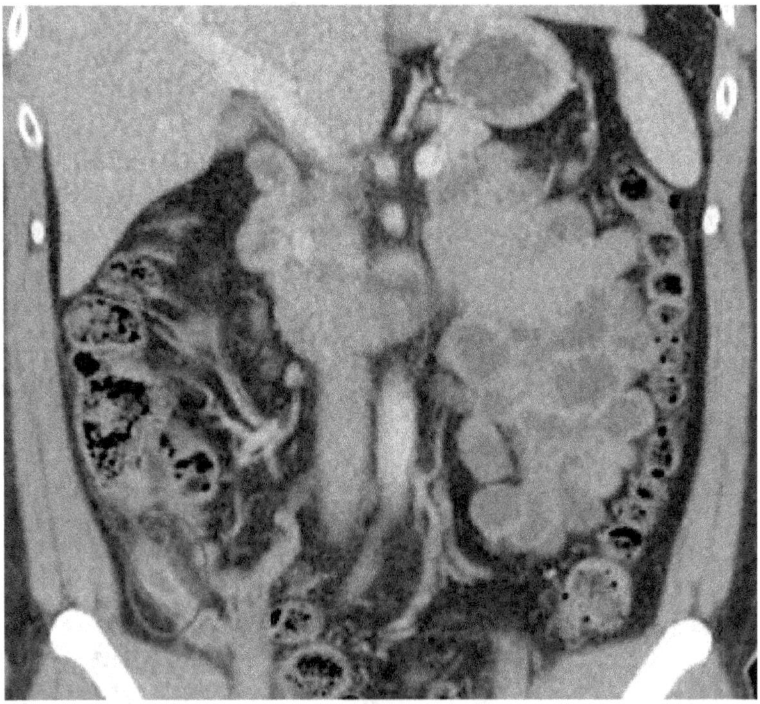

Figure 33. Coronal images show a thickened enhancing wall of the dilated appendix with adjacent fat stranding representing appendicitis.

If you suspect you might have appendicitis, it's important to seek medical attention right away. Your doctor may order a CT scan to take a closer look at your abdomen and confirm the diagnosis. Don't worry—getting a CT scan is a piece of cake (well, maybe not, but so much easier than a full-blown operation).

In most cases, appendicitis can be treated with surgery to remove the inflamed appendix. This specific type of surgery is called an appendectomy. It's a quick procedure, and you'll be back to your usual self in no time. Just think of it as getting rid of that annoying appendix, once and for all.

INTO THE BELLY

Free air is an emergency situation. This means that air is not located within the bowel, as it should be, so the bowel must have perforated or burst. Unless the reason for the air is a recent operation or a tube being placed, free air in the abdomen indicates that the bowel has ruptured, and the patient may have to go to the operating room to repair the hole in the bowel. Free air can be seen in *Figure 34* as the black that the arrow is pointing to, lying between the ribs and the liver.

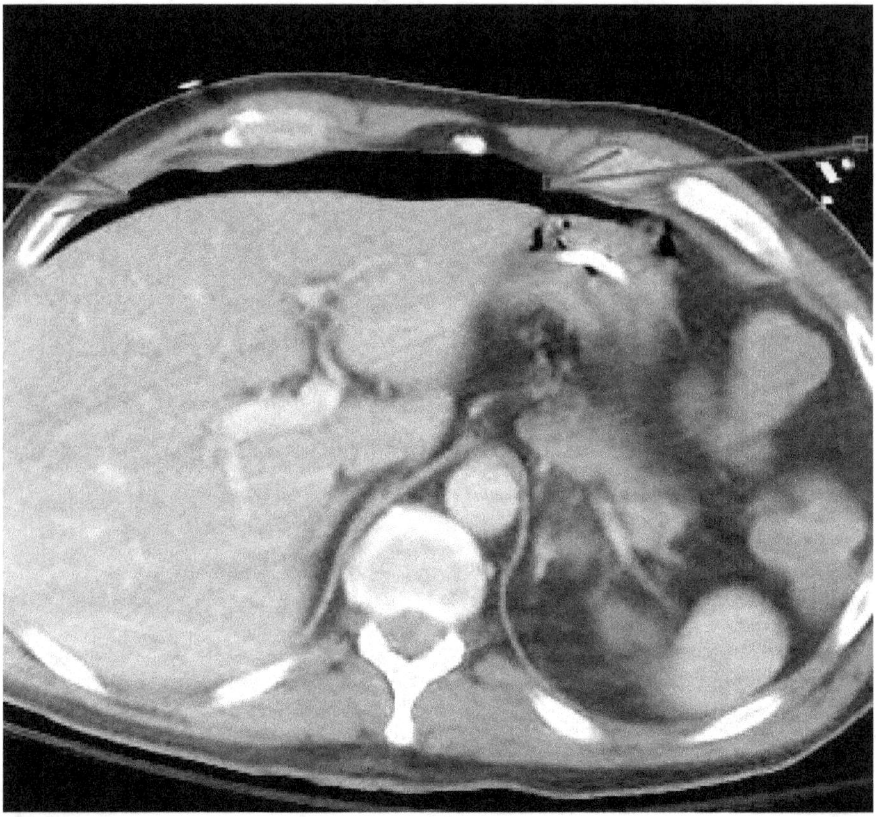

Figure 34. Axial image with arrows pointing to black within the upper abdomen which is the same appearance as air on the outside of the patient. Air within the abdomen that is not within bowel is called free air.

One reason for the bowel rupturing may be diverticulitis. **Diverticulitis** is a condition in which the colon becomes inflamed, resulting in an outpouching, a little protrusion (which usually develops from a lack of fiber in a diet). This can cause the bowel lumen to rupture; in *Figure 35*, only a few dots of air can be seen amidst the extensive inflammatory fat stranding. The fat is depicted in black on the scan; when fat becomes inflamed, it appears to be hazy and fuzzy, indicating irritation, which tells the radiologist that something is wrong.

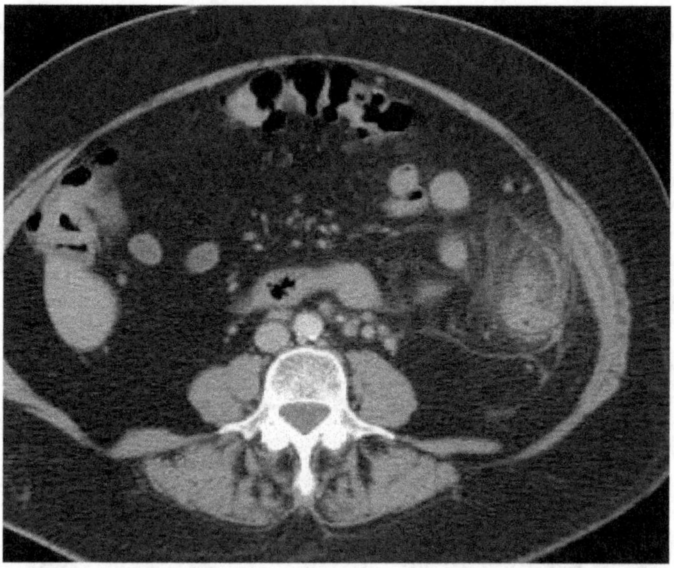

Figure 35. Circled is an area of fat stranding around a structure next to the left colon. This is a diverticulum – an outpouching of the colon- that has become inflamed, therefore called diverticulitis.

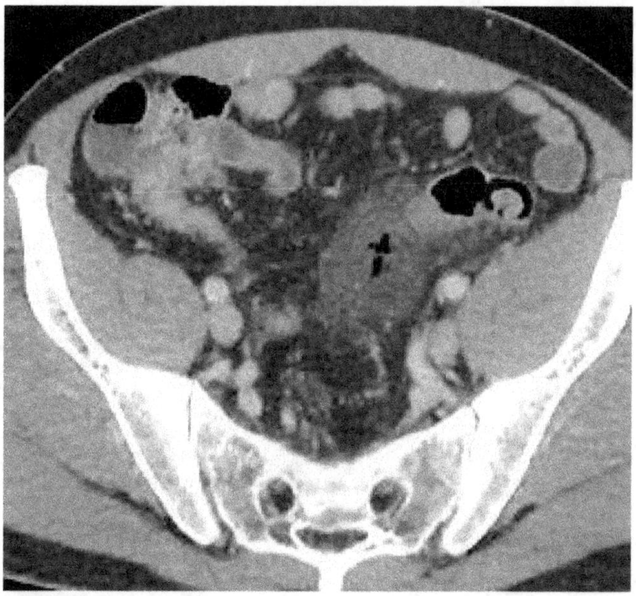

Figure 36.Circled is air (black) within the fat of the abdomen rather than within the bowel lumen. Adjacent fat stranding around a diverticulum is seen and this is a localized micro perforation from acute diverticulitis.

Figure 36 demonstrates another instance in which the bowel has ruptured just a little, which is called localized micro perforation. As it is very small, the doctors may treat the diverticulitis with antibiotics and hope that the hole seals up. If it gets worse, the patient may have to go to surgery.

CONCLUSIONS

So, there you have it—a glimpse into the wild world of abdominal diseases and how radiology plays a crucial role in diagnosing and treating them. Remember: our abdomens may be full of surprises but, with the help of CT scans, we can navigate through any digestive dilemma that comes our way.

CHAPTER 3

CHEST IMAGING AND DISEASES: PEEKING INSIDE THE CHEST

We will now be taking a peek inside the chest—not literally, of course, because that would require some serious cutting, and we're all about non-invasive imaging techniques here.

So, what exactly is hiding inside your chest? Well, besides your heart and lungs, there's a whole world of possibilities waiting to be discovered, with the help of CT scans. Think of it as a treasure chest—instead of gold and jewels, you might find a pesky little lung nodule or a sneaky rib fracture. Just remember: when it comes to radiology, the chest is like a mystery waiting to be solved. Each scan tells a unique story, whether it's a thrilling tale of pneumonia or a heartwarming saga of clear lungs and healthy organs. So, get ready to dive headfirst into the fascinating world of chest imaging.

THE LUNGS

We will first be speaking about the main organs of the respiratory system: the **lungs**, which are located on each side of the heart. The lungs give the body oxygen by completing a gas exchange and removing waste products, such as carbon dioxide; without the lungs, humans would not be able to breathe. The lungs resemble two cones.

To visualize the lungs, a function of the CT scanner (called window settings, which refers to the range and center point of the scan image) is helpful, as there is a specific mode for "lung windows". This enables the lungs themselves, including masses and lung diseases, to be evaluated, as seen in *Figure 37*. If this mode was not used, the lungs would not be imaged correctly—showing up as completely black on the regular windows used for seeing the abdominal organs, for example. So, it's like finding light at the end of the dark tunnel or switching the light on in a black hole. The right lung is made of three lobes, while the left is made of two lobes. *Figure 38* shows an axial slice through healthy lungs, with lung windows turned on.

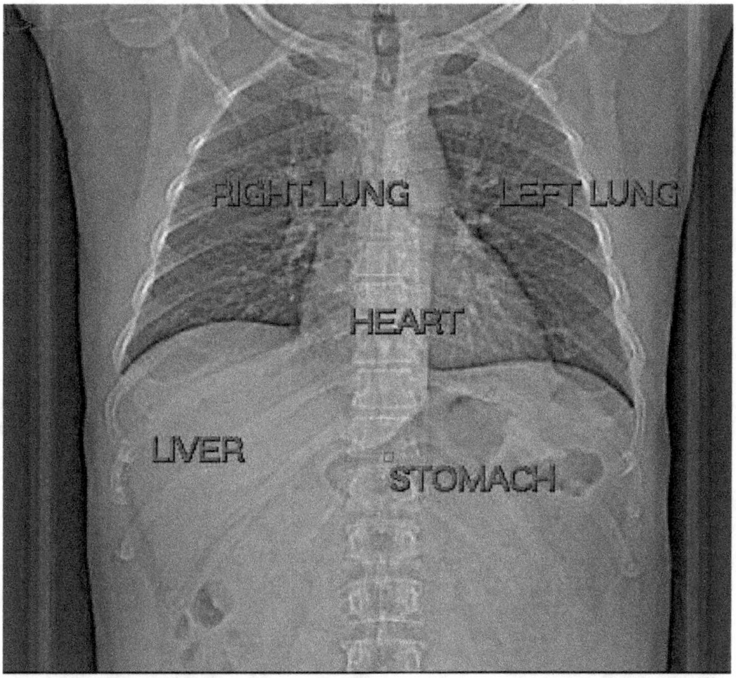

Figure 37. A CT scout view of the chest with labelled structures. This has a similar appearance to what a chest Xray would look like. This can be used to plan where the CT images will start and end.

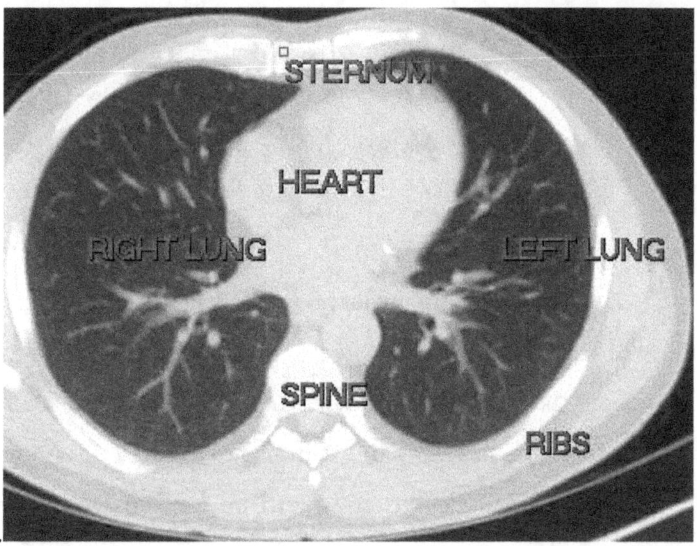

Figure 38. An axial CT with lung windows with the organs labelled.

LUNG ABNORMALITIES

We will now be diving into the realm of respiratory infections, starting with everyone's favorite lung ailment: **pneumonia**. Pneumonia is like the unwelcome guest that crashes your lung party and refuses to leave. It's caused by pesky bacteria or viruses sneaking into your lungs and setting up camp. Symptoms can include fever, coughing, and difficulty breathing.

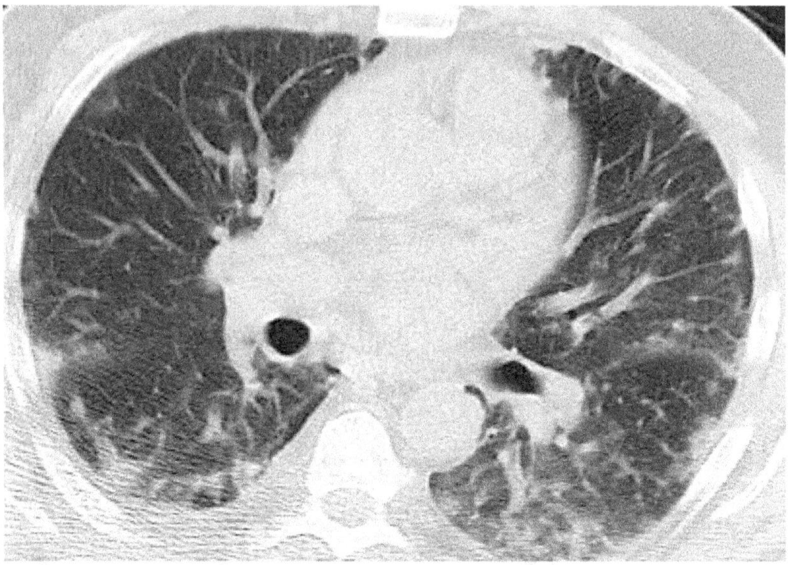

Figure 39. Patchy blobs around the outside of the lungs which one can almost see through (ground glass) is typical of COVID pneumonia.

People can develop pneumonia as a complication of the COVID-19 virus. *Figure 39* is an example of **COVID-19 pneumonia**, with peripheral ground glass opacities (gray areas on the CT scan that are seen in patients who have infections, inflammation, or diseases) that resemble the frosted glass of a shower stall. When COVID-19 pneumonia occurs, the lungs' air sacs become inflamed and fill with inflammatory cells, so we see these characteristic hazy, white patches on the peripheral (scattered on the border) of the scan.

Bacterial pneumonia's appearance is different when compared to that caused by COVID-19, as the white patches seen in a scan will be more solid than hazy. *Figure 40* is a good example of bacterial pneumonia: the white abnormalities, indicating infection or inflammation, are focal (in one spot) and are opaquer. The white patches now resemble a shower curtain, instead of frosted glass.

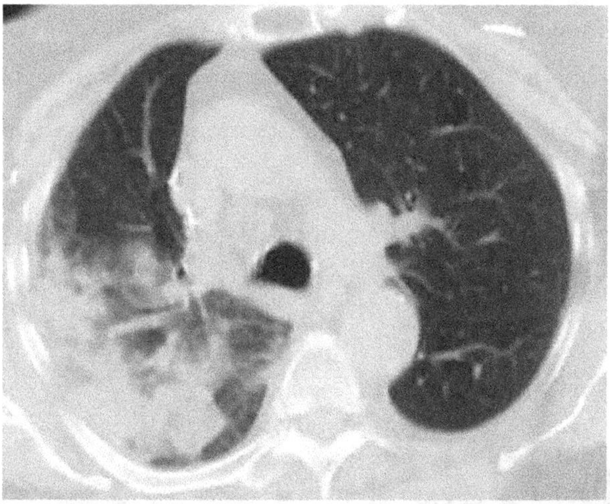

Figure 40. These patchy areas in the right lung are more dense/ whiter and one cannot see through them. This is called consolidation and is more typical of a bacterial pneumonia.

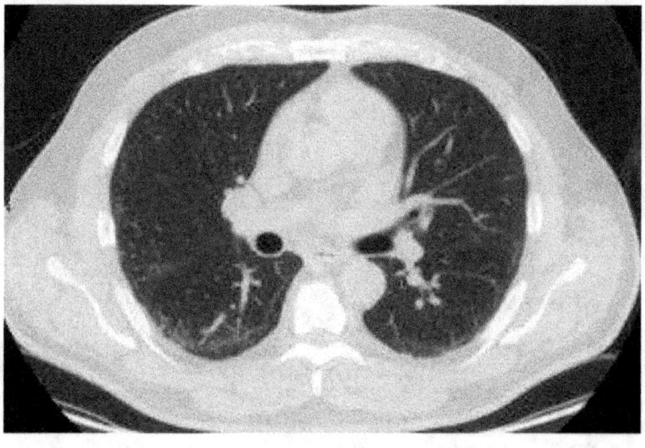

Figure 41. Axial CT shows the lungs to have cleared up following treatment of the pneumonia.

Figure 41 is a great example of the difference between the before and after of pneumonia. Now the lungs are clear!

However, pneumonia isn't the only respiratory infection that can wreak havoc on your lungs. There's also bronchitis, the annoying cousin of pneumonia that loves to hang out in your airways and make you cough up a storm. **Bronchi** are structures that transport air into and out of the lungs, which resemble tree-like branches on a CT scan. There are two main bronchi that lead into the lungs; as they move deeper within the lungs, they divide into smaller segments. **Bronchitis**, simply put, occurs when bronchial tubes or the airway in the lungs becomes inflamed (remember: "itis" means inflammation; hence, inflammation of the bronchi). This causes coughing due to mucus production in the bronchi, rather than air. *Figure 42* depicts lungs affected by both bronchitis and emphysema.

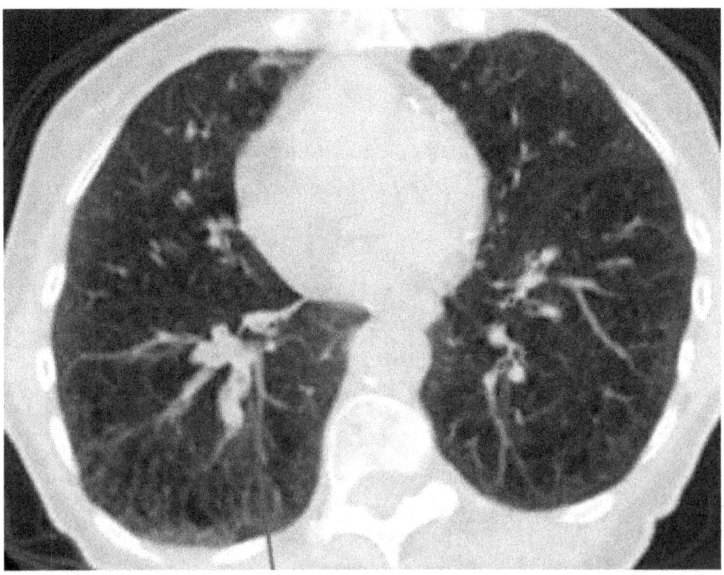

Figure 42. The arrow points to density(white) within the tubular bronchi - the airways that are meant to have air(black). These are filled with mucus and can make breathing difficult.

Emphysema is a lung disease usually caused by smoking, which results in destruction of the airways. In *Figure 43*, you will see tiny black holes in the lungs; these are not present in healthy lungs and represent the alveoli which are damaged. The alveoli are important, because they are the means by which the lungs and blood exchange oxygen and carbon dioxide, allowing us to breathe.

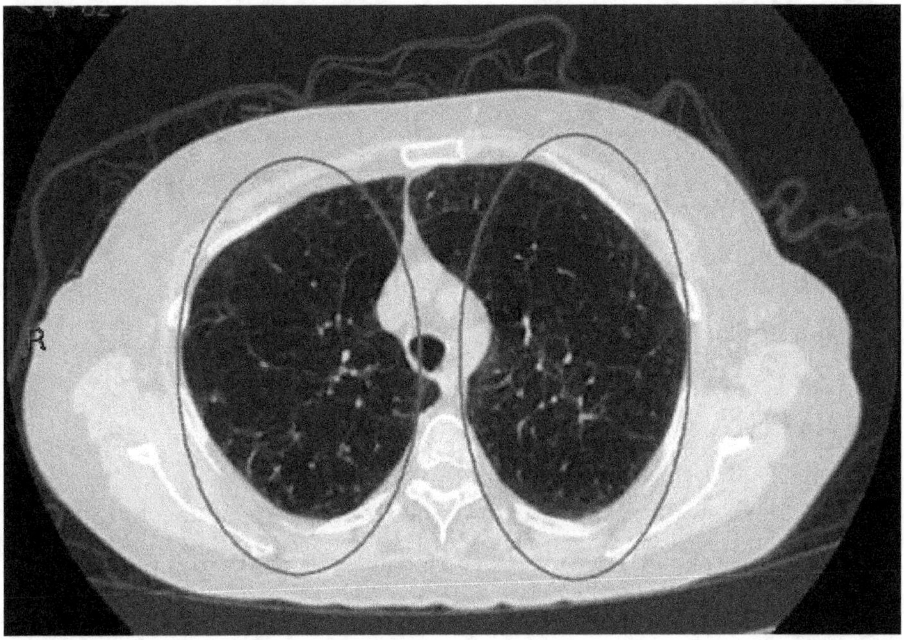

Figure 43. Circled are the lungs which contain multiple holes. This is the destroyed lung parenchyma that are typical of emphysema.

Compare the lungs in *Figure 43* with the normal lungs in *Figure 44*.

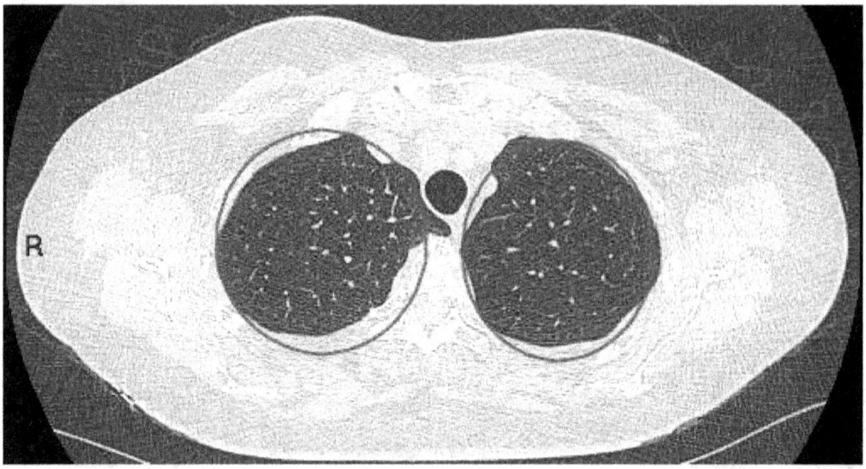

Figure 44. Circled is an axial CT image with lung windows showing normal lungs with no cysts/areas of alveolar destruction.

You want to keep your lungs healthy, so no smoking or vaping—it's just not cool!

THE HEART

The next step on our journey is located between the lungs in the middle of the chest. The **heart** beats around 60–100 times per minute...; with each beat, the heart pumps blood, which carries oxygen to all over the body. It also carries waste products, such as carbon dioxide, back to the lungs to be removed through gas exchange, with oxygen taken in by inspiration and carbon dioxide taken out of the body by expiration. The heart does not look as it is often pictured in popular culture; instead, it is roughly the same shape and size as a man's closed fist. Within the heart are two atria (the right and left atrium), as well as two ventricles (right ventricle and left ventricle).

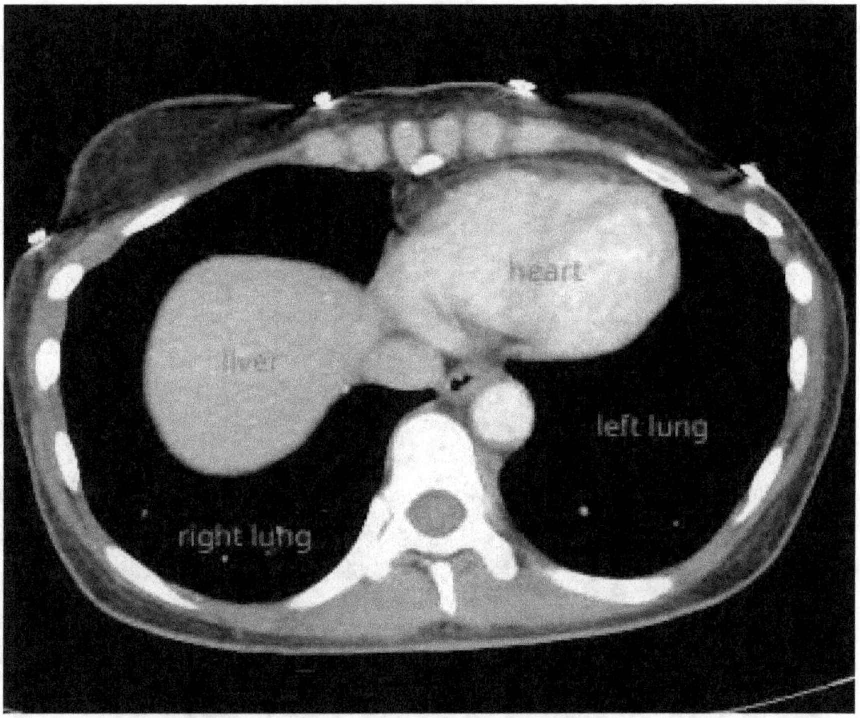

Figure 45. An axial CT with mediastinal windows. The lungs appear black. This is for assessment of the other structures in the chest.

THE PULMONARY ARTERIES

The **pulmonary arteries** are a pair of blood vessels that carry oxygen-poor blood from the heart to the lungs to become oxygenated again through gas exchange and the removal of waste products, like carbon dioxide. This is an important function, as the body needs an equally distributed supply of oxygen to live. Sometimes (luckily, not very often!), blood clots travel to the lungs, which can interfere with gas exchange. When a blood clot is very large and extends along the main left and right pulmonary arteries, it is called a **saddle pulmonary embolism**. As seen in *Figure 46*, there is a darker grey that straddles the pulmonary artery, where it splits into the right and left branches. The main pulmonary artery is circled, which splits into the left pulmonary artery (the oval circle on the left) and the right pulmonary artery (the oval circle next to the arrow). The clot fills the entire right pulmonary artery and extends into part of the left pulmonary artery. When clots are large and blood thinners cannot cure them, a certain type of radiologist—called interventional radiologists—must remove the clots. Clots are also called thrombus/thrombi, which is why this procedure is called a thrombectomy.

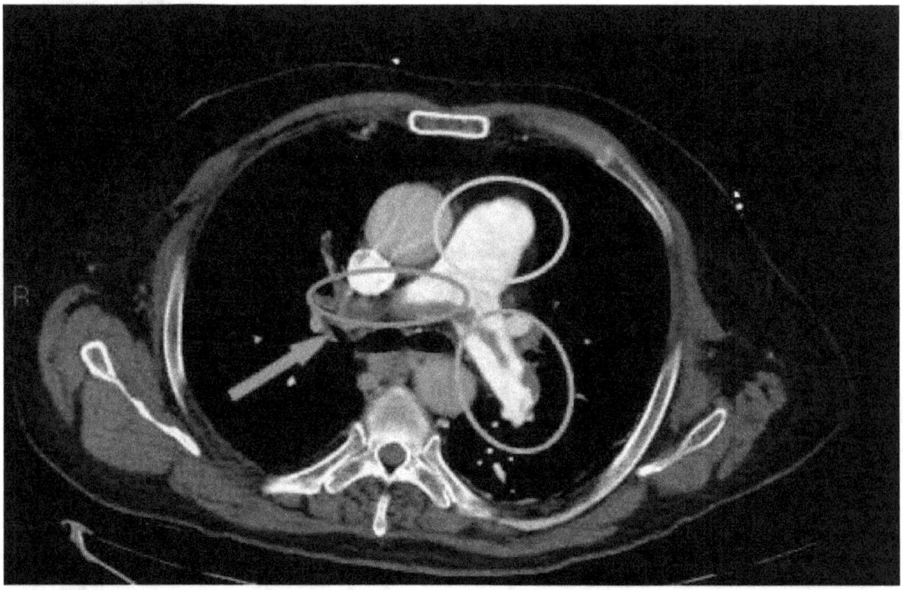

Figure 46. The white is contrast which should be filling up the pulmonary arteries. The arrow points to grey within the white that straddles the pulmonary artery from right to left and this is called a saddle pulmonary embolism.

In *Figure 47*, you will see a trail of grey following the pulmonary artery into the right lung. The grey, which is circled, is the clot; the white in the image represents the contrast moving within the healthy blood vessels, which is what we want to see, as it indicates the blood is freely flowing.

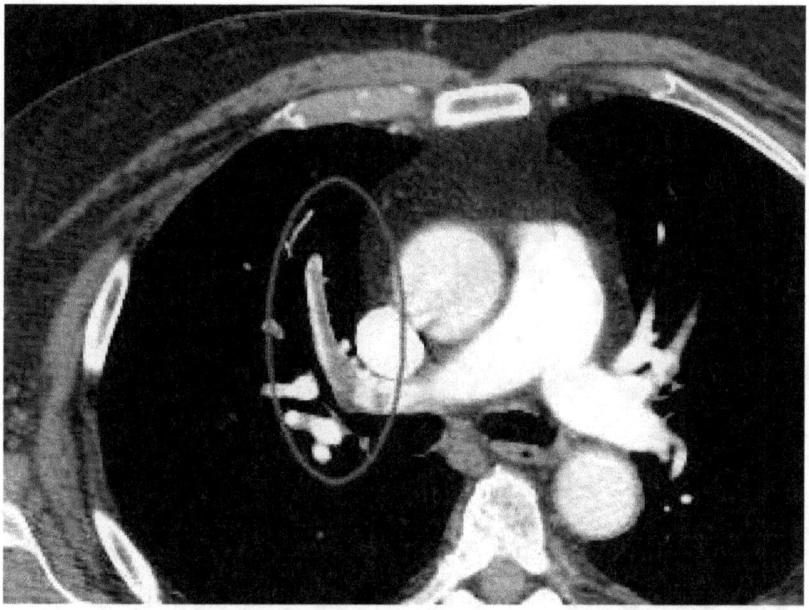

Figure 47. A small branch in the right upper lobe has grey filling defects within what is meant to be a white branch of the pulmonary artery to the right upper lobe of the lung.

Now, let's talk about the other major vessel in the chest. The largest artery in the body is called the **aorta**, which begins at the left ventricle of the heart and extends upwards to the chest, forming an arch. It provides blood flow to all the organs.

THE AORTA

The walls of the aorta are made of multiple circular layers. If the interior of one of the walls rips, the loose flap of tissue can block blood flow and cause a clot. This clot can get so big that it can block the flow to the aorta, which is the biggest blood vessel in your body and can cause death. In the example in *Figure 48*, the aorta has flow in the false and true lumen. The true lumen is where blood flow is normal, whereas the false lumen is blood going through the hole in the wall that is torn.

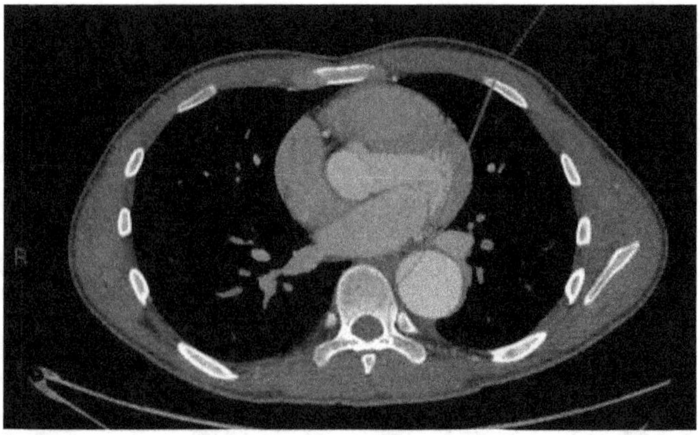

Figure 48. Axial CT with mediastinal windows with the arrow pointing to a thin line called a dissection flap within the descending thoracic aorta.

An **aneurysm** is when any part of the blood vessels dilates. In this case, the aorta is dilated and aneurysmal. The flap of the torn aorta creates a line of tissue that divides the separate layers of the wall of the blood vessel, which creates an extra channel called the false lumen; blood can then fill this channel and enter the wall of the aorta, rather than in the true lumen, where the blood is meant to travel (i.e., contained within the walls of the blood vessel).

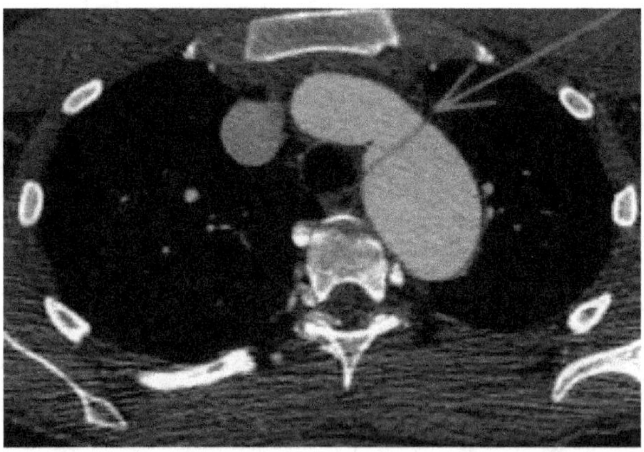

Figure 49. The thin dissection flap is seen within the aortic arch and beyond this the aorta has become more dilated than proximal to it, so this is called aneurysmal dilatation.

THE DIAPHRAGM

PNEUMOTHORAX

Pneumothorax is the abnormal collection of air in the space next to the lungs, which called pleural space (the cavity between the lungs and underneath the chest wall). If this air collection gets too big, it can squash the lungs and heart and lead to a lack of oxygen. In *Figure 50*, the black space, which is not meant to be present in that area, represents air surrounding the lung, making it look as if the lung is floating.

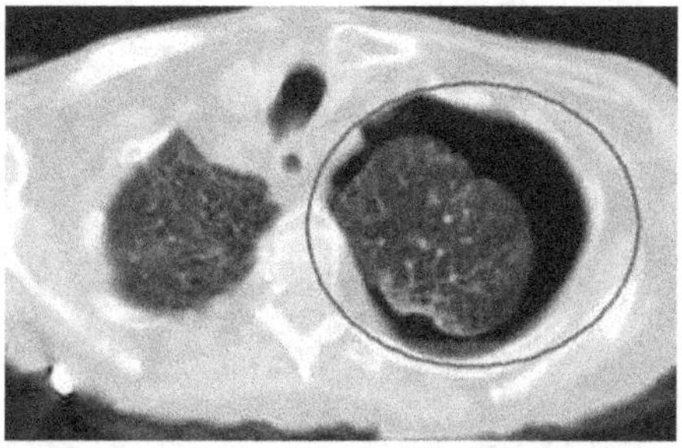

Figure 50. Circled is the left lung. With lung windows the lung parenchyma can be seen in the center circled by the air that is black that lies within the pleural space.

To fix a pneumothorax, the radiologist inserts a tube into the patient to suck out the air, which is pictured in *Figure 51*.

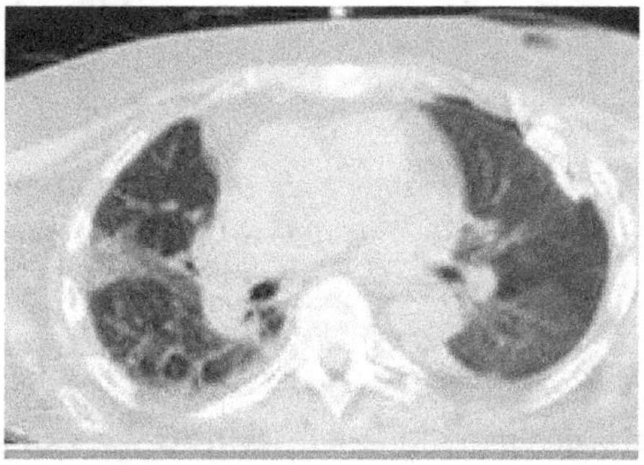

Figure 51. A white structure in the anterior aspect of the left lung with a coiled tip is a pigtail catheter that has been inserted into the air of the pleural space to suck out the air and leave the left lung re-expanded.

Figure 52 is an example of a tension pneumothorax, which has shifted the heart to the left side and pushed the diaphragm down. It is abnormal for the right side of the diaphragm to be so black (i.e., lacking any visible lines representing the vessels passing through it); instead, it should look more like the left side, where vessels can be seen, pictured in white. The black C-shaped form, visible on the scan around the collapsed right lung, is excessive air which is an emergency.

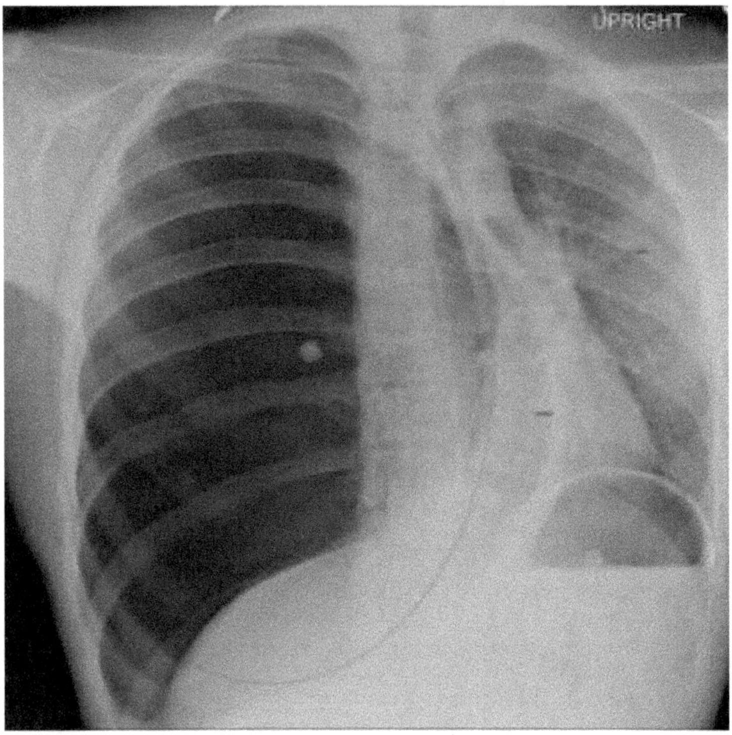

Figure 52. Chest Xray shows a large right pneumothorax with shift of the heart and mediastinum to the left so the large amount of air compresses on these structures which can compromise their function. This is an emergency called a tension pneumothorax.

Luckily, the radiologist, like a superhero, can insert a chest tube—circled on *Figure 52* as it enters through the right chest wall—which has nicely re-expanded the right lung.

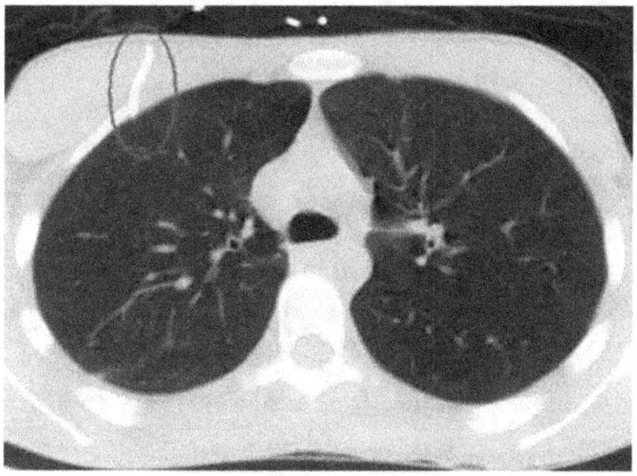

Figure 53. Circled is the entry of the white line that represents a pigtail catheter that was inserted and expanded the lung to normal size expelling the air that was in the pleural space.

The same person's CT scan, after the right chest tube was placed, has a whole different appearance, as seen in *Figure 53.* The lungs and heart are back in their normal locations. The chest tube is circled in the right upper chest in *Figure 54.* It looks like a whole different person—almost back to health!

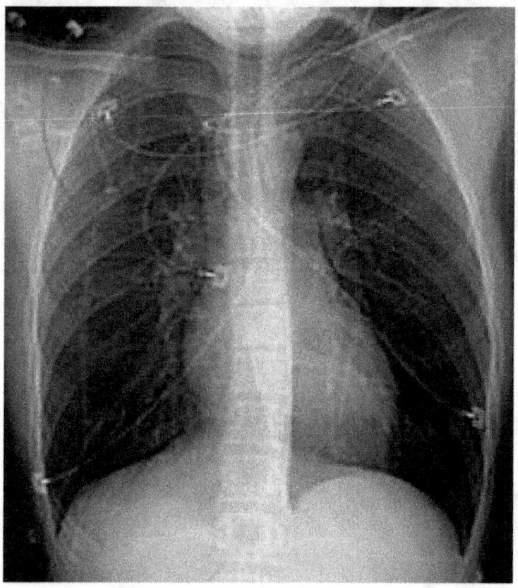

Figure 54. CT scout view showing the catheter circled as it enters the right chest/pleural space.

Let's now talk about when something other than air fills up the space around the lungs.

HEMOTHORAX

Hemothorax is when the pleural space fills with blood, rather than air. *Figure 55* represents a large hemothorax in the right side. The higher densities—that is, the lighter grey within the areas of grey fluid—represent areas filled with blood.

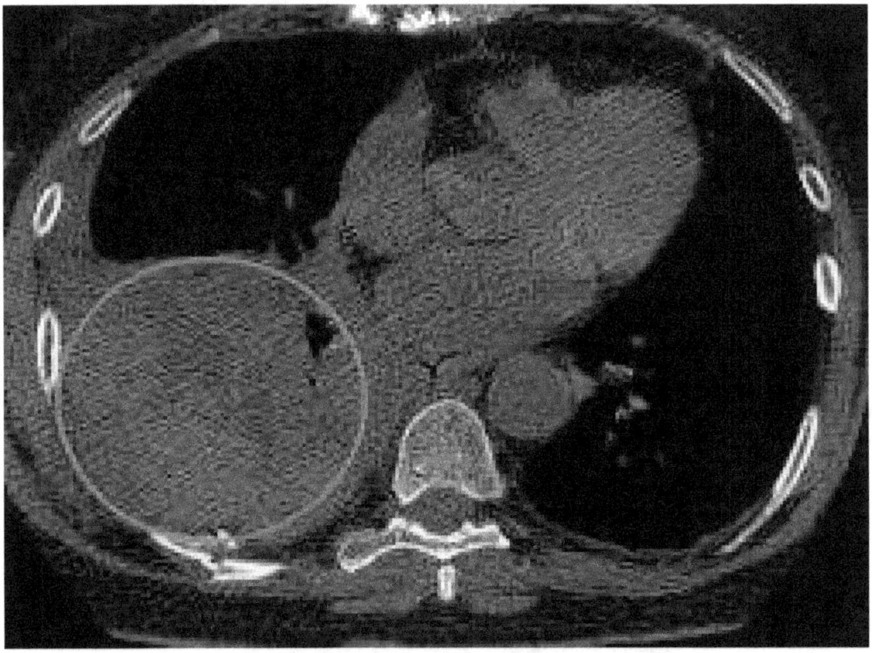

Figure 55. Circled is heterogenous grey appearance to the right lung which represents mixed densities/ ages of blood.

RIB FRACTURE

A **rib fracture** is when the rib bone breaks. There are cracks in the broken rib, compared to the normal rib that is fully pieced together. Circled in *Figure 55* is an example of what a fractured rib looks like.

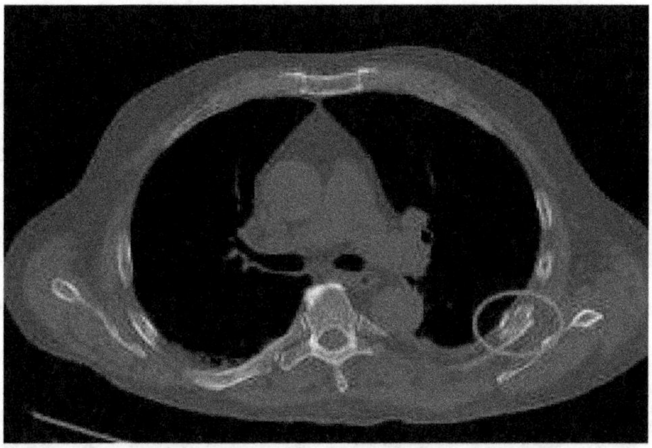

Figure 56. Circled is a left posterior rib fracture with multiple parts so called a comminuted fracture.

When it comes to imaging the heart, blood vessels and lungs, CT scans are like the crusaders of the radiology world. They can give us detailed pictures of the lungs and the heart's structure thereby helping doctors to diagnose and treat cardiovascular diseases with precision. Just imagine it as a high-tech peek inside your chest, without the need for any invasive procedures.

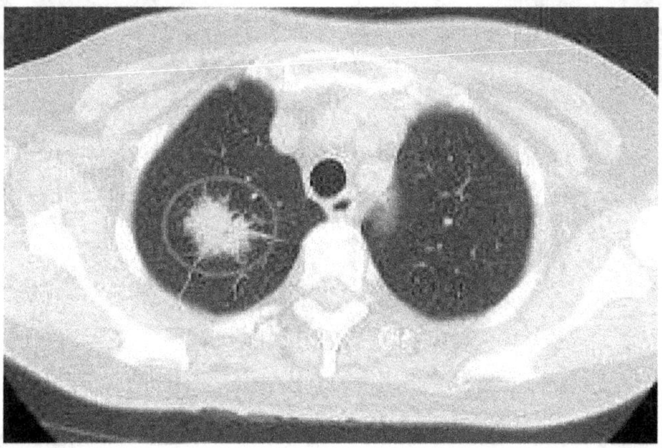

Figure 57. Axial CT of the chest shows a very irregularly marginated right lung mass that is the typical appearance of a lung cancer.

LUNG CANCER

Lung cancer is when there is a spiculated(spiky) or irregularly marginated mass. *Figure 57* displays a large white spiky mass that is not meant to be there. If you have lung cancer, that is bad news, and you might need to see a cancer doctor fast! A few of the causes of lung cancer are smoking, second hand smoke and air pollution. It is important to not increase the risk of getting lung cancer so don't smoke!

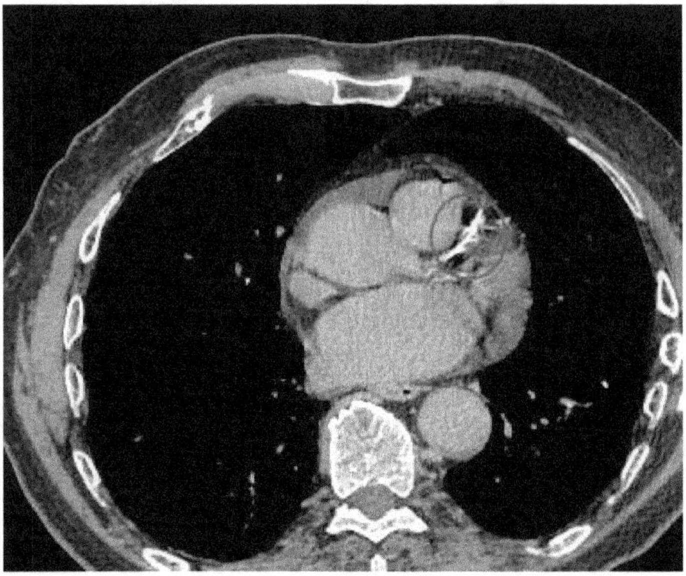

Figure 58. Circled is a white line which represents extensive calcification along one of the coronary arteries- in this case the left anterior descending coronary artery.

CORONARY CALCIFICATION

Coronary calcification is when the heart arteries get calcified meaning there is calcium in the coronary artery, one of the blood vessels feeding the heart. If the arteries have too much calcium in the blood vessel wall, this would cause narrowing. Therefore, the amount of blood going through to the heart is decreased, which could eventually lead to a heart attack. The risk is increased in smokers and people who have unhealthy diets, including eating fatty foods, which are rich in cholesterol, as well as individuals who have increased stress or blood pressure. It is important to pay attention to our heart health early on and make smart choices like eating healthy, staying active, and not stressing too much about that math test.

In conclusion, the heart may be a mysterious and sometimes finicky organ, but with the help of radiology, we can navigate the world of cardiovascular diseases with confidence. So, let's put on our imaginary lab coats, grab our virtual stethoscopes, and embark on a journey to keep our hearts happy and healthy. Remember, laughter is the best medicine, but a good CT scan comes in a close second.

CHAPTER 4

BRAIN IMAGING AND DISEASES: UNRAVELING THE MYSTERIES OF THE BRAIN

We are now going to dive deep into the intricate complexities of the brain – that squishy, mysterious organ inside your head that controls everything from your thoughts to your movements. Let's get ready to unravel the mysteries of the brain!

Did you know that the human brain is made up of billions of nerve cells called neurons? These neurons communicate with each other through electrical impulses, forming intricate networks that allow you to think, feel, and experience the world around you. It's like a supercharged computer inside your head – only it doesn't come with a user manual!

When it comes to imaging the brain, radiologists use advanced techniques like CT scans to get a closer look at its inner workings. These scans provide detailed images of the brain's structure, allowing doctors to diagnose conditions like tumors, strokes, and brain injuries. It's like peeking behind the curtain of your own mind – but without the need for any magic tricks!

But beware – the brain is a tricky beast! It's prone to all sorts of weird malfunctions, from migraines to memory loss. Just know when you forget where you left your phone or struggle to concentrate in class, remember that it's all part of the brain's quirky charm. Embrace the chaos, and who knows – you might just unlock the secrets of the universe!

Let's start with the basics. The brain is the most complex part of the body. It's like the mastermind behind the way you move and speak, how you absorb and retain information, and what you think and feel. All of what we do and how we perform actions in our daily life are controlled by the brain including the digestion of our foods and beating of our hearts.

The **cerebral cortex** is in the outer parts of the brain and consists of many folds causing the well-known wrinkled appearance. It is made of cortical grey matter which is lighter than the more internal white matter of the brain on a CT scan. As you can see circled on either side of the midline, the white matter is seemingly darker than the grey matter which is confusing because you would think it would be the opposite! The function of the **grey matter** is receiving information and regulating outgoing information whereas the **white matter** transmits signals to other regions of the brain, spinal cord, and body. The black stuff is **cerebral spinal fluid (CSF)** or the lubricant which surrounds the brain, so the brain lives comfortably. CSF goes into the ventricles which channel the fluid into the spinal canal which is also surrounded by fluid.

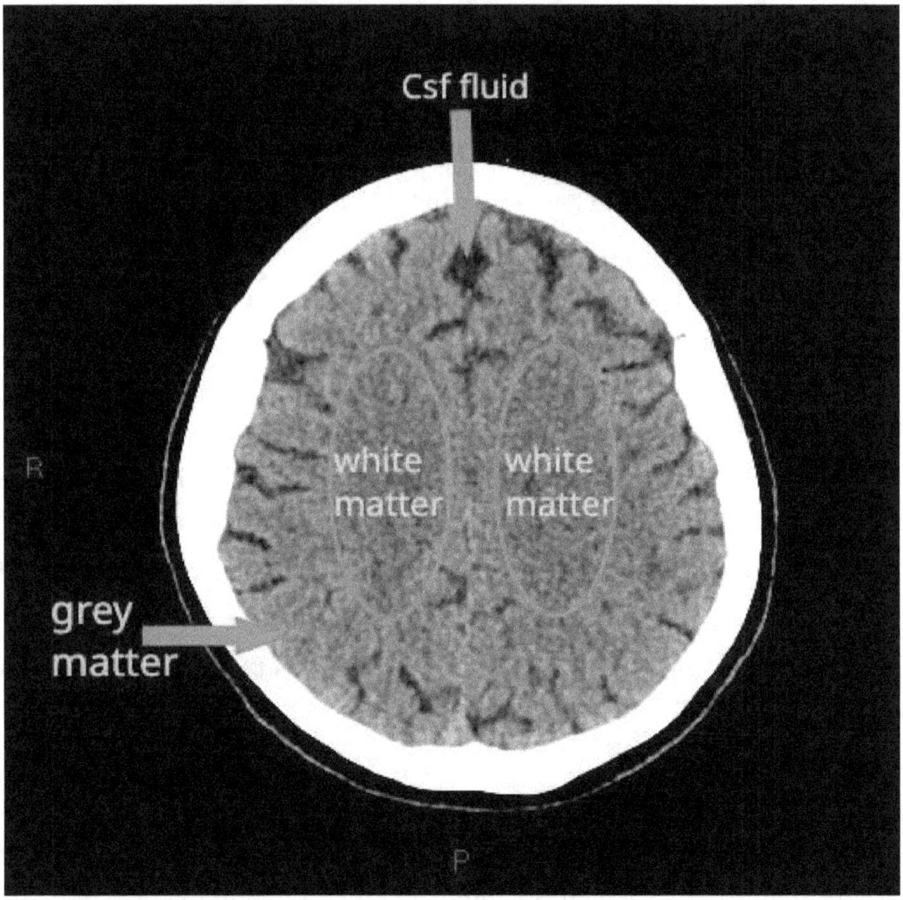

Figure 59. An axial image of the brain with parts of the brain parenchyma, substance of the solid component of the brain, and cerebrospinal fluid (CSF) labelled.

As we slice from top to bottom of the brain, more parts of the brain are visible. In *Figure 60* we see the **frontal lobes** which are responsible for higher cognitive functions such as voluntary movements, problem solving, organization, memory, and control of personal interaction. They are the largest lobes in the brain and are important because they are the ones allowing you to learn all the information in this book right as we speak. Circled in the front are the **basal ganglia**. The modulation of force, amplitude, and speed of movement is facilitated by the basal ganglia. The **occipital lobes** are on the bottom section of the brain, and they are what are in control of visual perception including color, form, and motion.

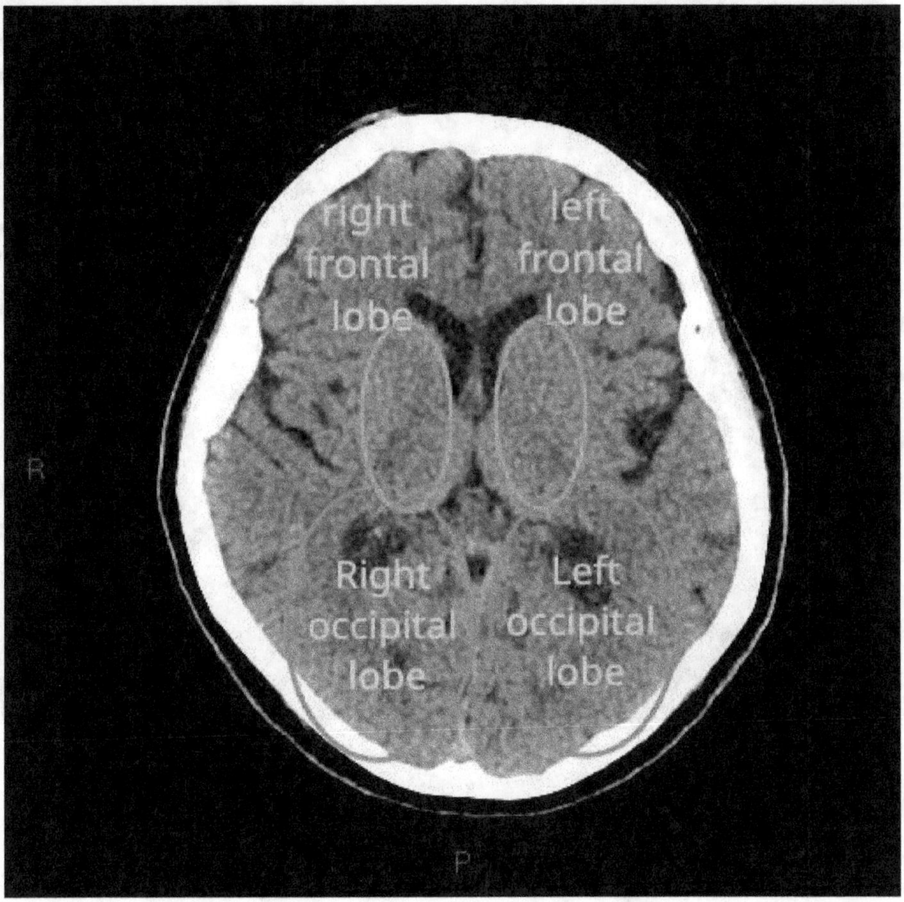

Figure 60. An axial image further down at the level of the frontal horns of the ventricles. The circles that are not labelled in the center represent the basal ganglia which are major control centers of the brain.

The **sylvian fissure**, a wide fissure that divides the temporal lobe from the frontal and parietal lobes, contains the **insula** which forms the inner surface of the cerebral cortex.

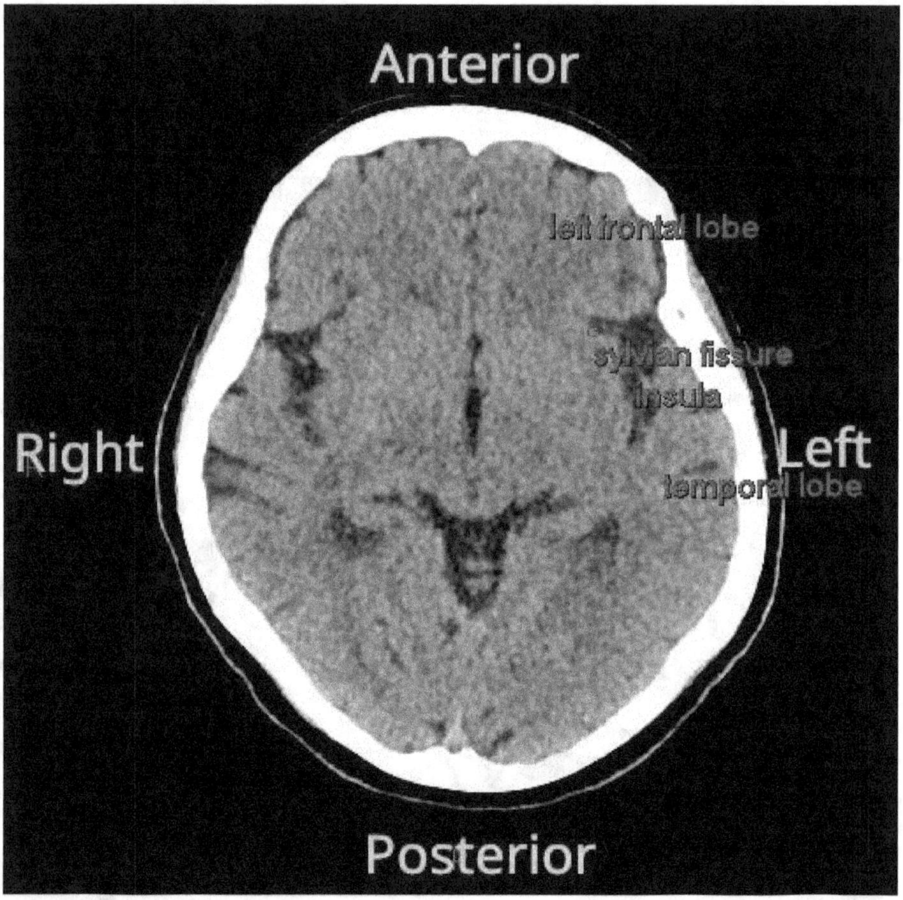

Figure 61. An image at the level of the sylvian fissure which separates the frontal and temporal lobes is where the insula lives.

The loss of definition of the insular cortex, as you will see later may be an early sign of an acute infarct of the middle cerebral artery territory. In *Figure 61*, however, the brain is normal. Additionally, something you might need to know is how to name the other sides of the body besides right and left. Anterior is used to speak of the front, which you can recall because the Latin definition of ante is front, and posterior means back, which is also easy to remember because the prefix, post, is often associated with after or end.

The **temporal lobes** are on both sides of the brain, as the brain is symmetrical.

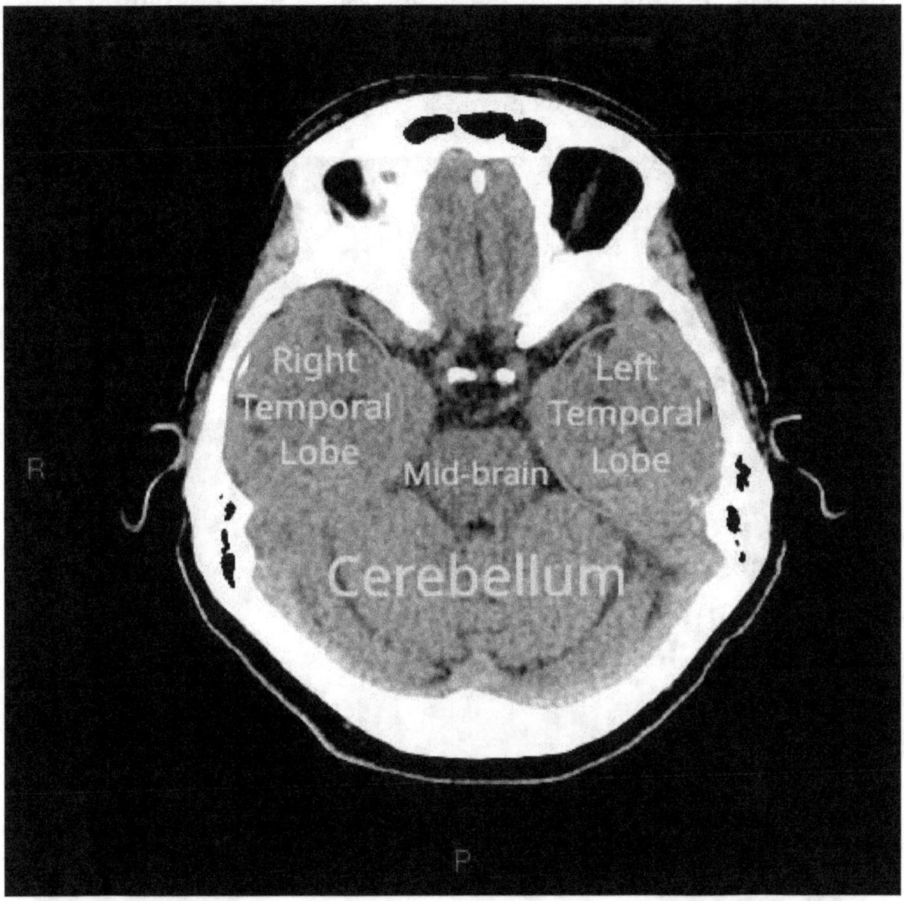

Figure 62. An axial CT slice slightly lower in the brain where the middle cranial fossa and the posterior fossa lies.

The purpose of the **temporal lobes** are to understand and respond to the world around us, by using our senses. These are located behind the ears and are the second largest lobes besides the frontal lobes. The **mid-brain** is situated at the top of the brainstem and underneath the cerebral cortex, in the middle area of the brain. The midbrain is a component of the central nervous system and plays a crucial role in processing auditory and visual information as well as in motor movement, especially eye movements. In the area of the brain between the midbrain and the back of the skull is called the **cerebellum**, which stands for "little brain". It is shaped like a heart and its role is to control and coordinate muscle movement.

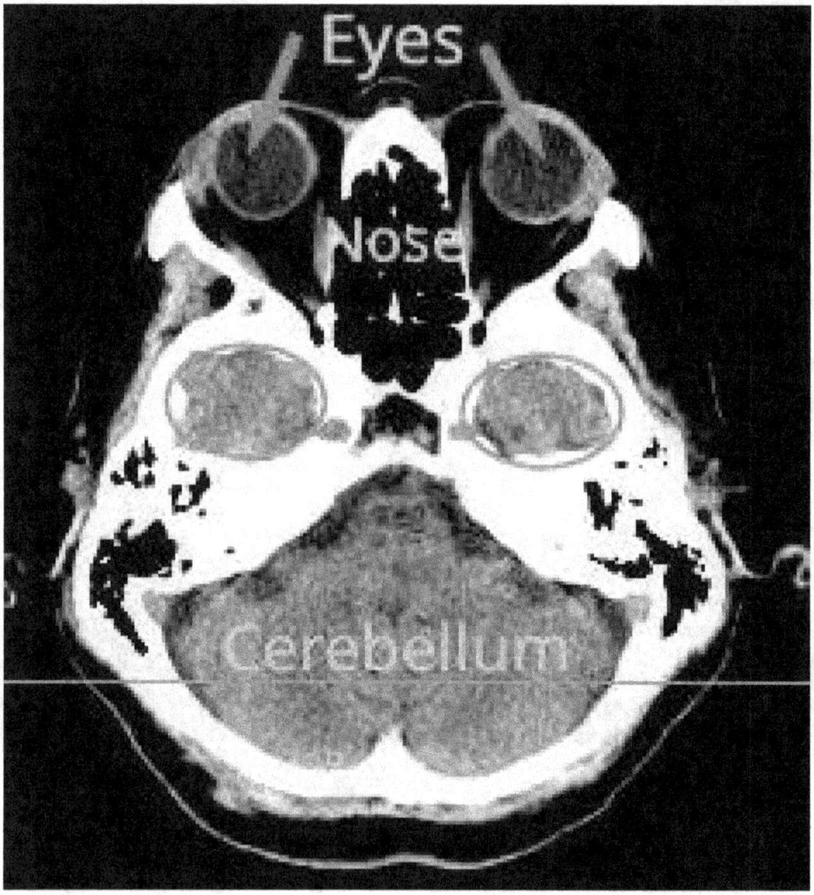

Figure 63. Axial CT slice more inferior at the level of the eyes and nose.

This is one of the lower slices of the brain where we can see the eyes and nose that give us the ability to see and breathe. Circled are the temporal lobes that are still visible and the heart shaped cerebellum on the posterior of the brain.

Understanding Stroke

Ah, the mysterious world of strokes. No, we're not talking about the kind you use to paint a masterpiece or hit a golf ball. We're talking about the kind that can happen in your brain, causing all sorts of chaos.

First things first, what exactly is a stroke? Well, remember how I said the brain is like a super important control center for your body? Now, imagine a traffic jam happening in your brain because a blood vessel gets blocked or bursts. That's basically what a stroke is – a traffic jam in your brain due to a blockage of a blood vessel that can wreak havoc on your body.

Now, you might be wondering, "How can I avoid getting stuck in this brain traffic jam?" The key is to keep your blood vessels healthy and happy. That means eating right, exercising, and not smoking (unless you want your blood vessels to throw a tantrum and cause a stroke).

But wait, there's more! Did you know that strokes can come in different flavors? Yep, there are actually two main types of strokes: **ischemic strokes** and **hemorrhagic strokes**. Ischemic strokes happen when a blood vessel gets blocked, kind of like a clogged drain in your brain. Hemorrhagic strokes, on the other hand, occur when a blood vessel bursts, causing blood to leak into your brain (yikes!).

ISCHEMIC STROKES

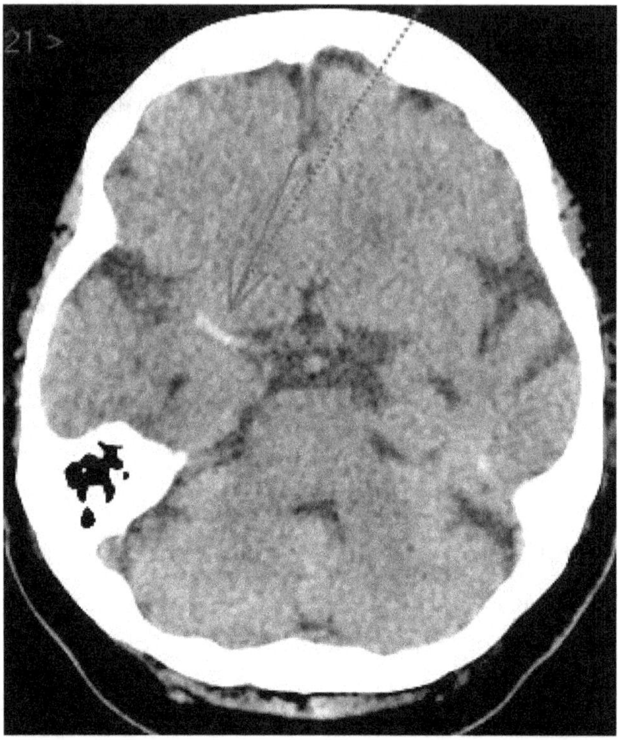

Figure 63. Axial CT at the level of the sylvian fissures where the middle cerebral artery lives. The right middle cerebral artery is dense (white) compared to the left which cannot be seen as it is like the adjacent brain parenchyma. This is called the "hyperdense MCA sign".

Hyperdense middle cerebral artery (MCA) - Hyperdense means that something is too white. In this case a blood clot is in the right middle cerebral artery, the line at which the arrow is pointing, which is white, meaning it is more hyperdense than the opposite side. Remember that the brain is supposed to be symmetrical. The clot causes there to be no flow to the right side of the brain which means that the person is experiencing a stroke. This vessel supplies the right part of the brain but controls the left side of the body. That would mean the patient comes in with left facial droop, left arm weakness, and left leg weakness. In other words when the blood flow to the brain is on one side, the opposite side is the one that gets affected.

When contrast/dye is given (*Figure 64*) one can see that the left side MCA (Name B02) lights up with flow of blood in that region, but the vessel is not seen on the right side (Name: B01), because it is blocked.

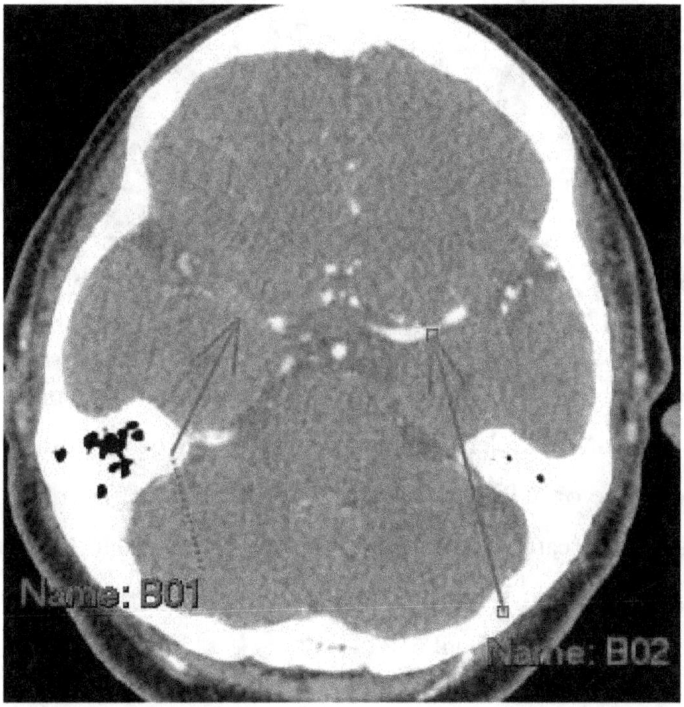

Figure 64. Axial CT image of a CT angiogram where contrast fills the vessels demonstrates no contrast in the region of the right middle cerebral artery as it is blocked. The left middle cerebral artery labelled B02 has contrast filling it so is white and normal.

In this next example (*Figure 65*), the left side is affected as there is ill definition of the sylvian fissure compared to the right side where the fissure can be seen. Additionally, edema(swelling) of the left brain is visible which is a sign of stroke.

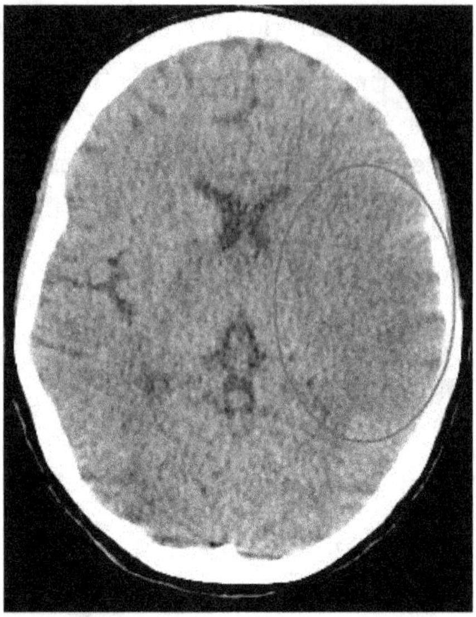

Figure 65. Axial noncontrast CT shows blurring of the junction of the grey and white matter on the left, a sign of early infarction/stroke.

Strokes are much more easily identified with a specific imaging sequence on MRI called diffusion weighted images. Diffusion-weighted MRI is a type of MRI that uses water molecule diffusion, which is then processed to create contrast in the images. This imaging sequence is also more sensitive and specific for detecting acute stroke when compared with CT and conventional MRI.

This is beautifully demonstrated in *Figure 66* of a **left posterior middle cerebral artery infarct**. The infarct can faintly be seen as a subtle grayer ill definition on CT, but when diffusion-weighted MRI is performed, a much more obvious abnormality is visible that even a kindergartener can point out. This technique employs diffusion to demonstrate how the stroke area lights up when the water molecules there are unable to move as quickly. So, if there is suspicion for a stroke and the CT is not very clear as to whether the suspicion is true, then an MRI can help definitively answer the question.

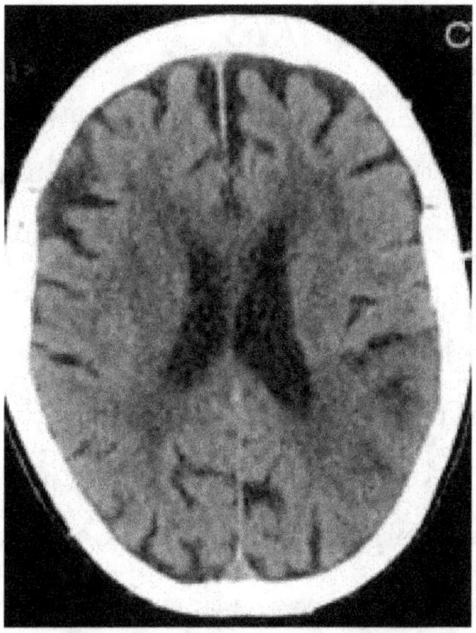

Figure 66. Axial CT of a different patient showing blurring of the left posterior brain which is subtle.

This is the same left posterior MCA infarct, but it is much more obvious and brighter on MRI diffusion sequence (*Figure 67*). See here the stroke is so much easier to spot because it is lightened up! Thank you, MRI!

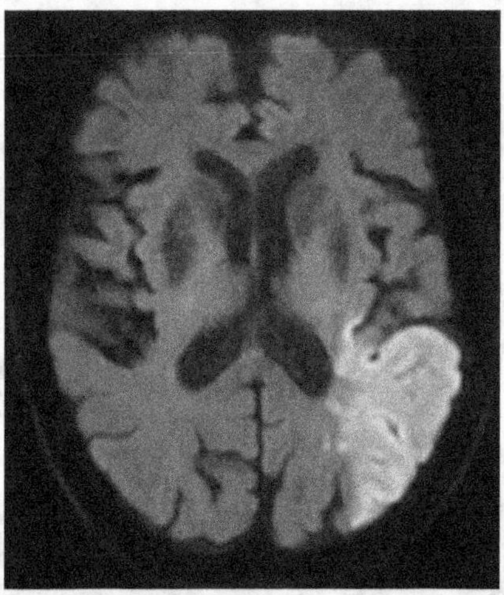

Figure 67. Diffusion weighted image of the same patient as the CT above shows the left middle cerebral artery infarct affecting the left parietal region as a bright area of restricted diffusion.

HEMORRHAGIC STROKES

Small left thalamic hemorrhage - As you can see there is a large white dot (circled) in the basil ganglia area as the thalamus is a part of the basil ganglia, shown in *Figure 73*. A small portion, as pointed out by the arrow, extends into the ventricles. What is important to remember is when there is bright white signal, we must be concerned that it may be blood. It is crucial to catch the hemorrhage early so it can be observed to make sure it does not get bigger and compromise the brain function. The patient may need surgery if the size is too large.

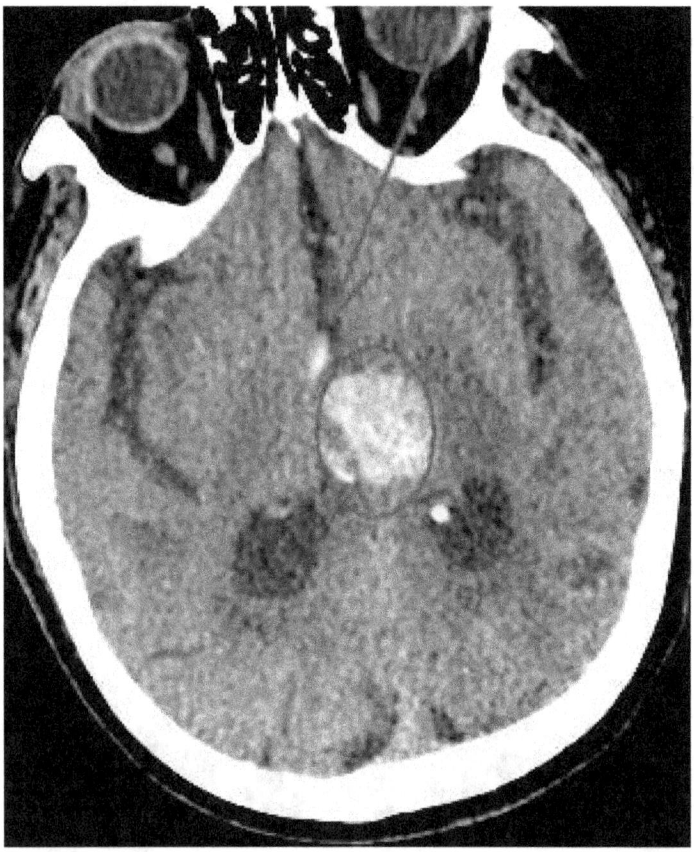

Figure 68. The circle demonstrates blood within the left thalamus. The arrow points to a small amount of blood extending into the adjacent ventricle.

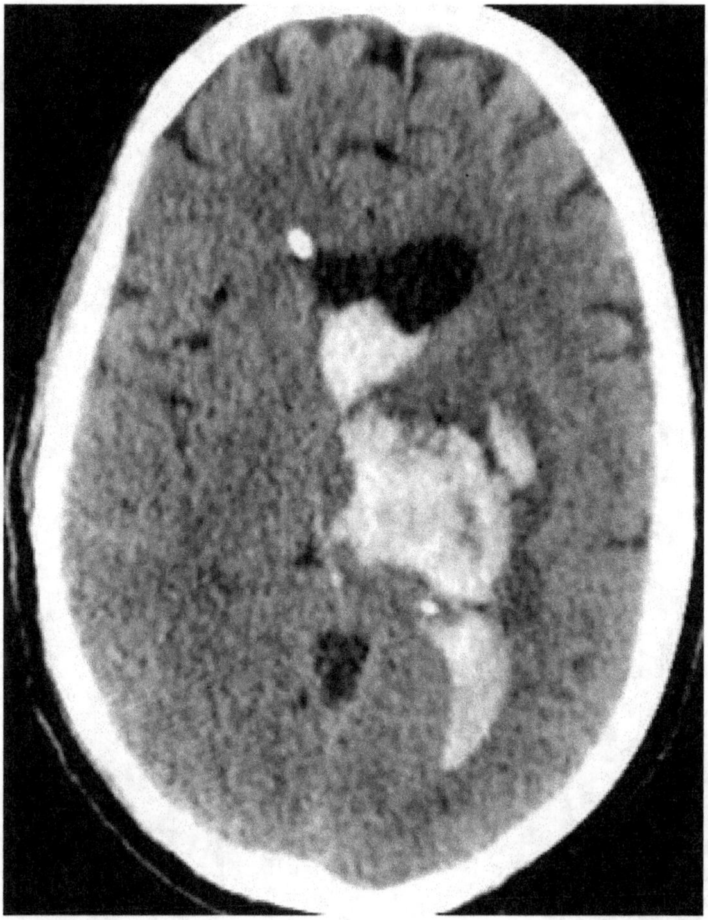

Figure 69. Below is a larger area of hemorrhage in the left basal ganglia extending into the ventricles. The blood blocks free flow of the CSF and causes hydrocephalus.

A **hemorrhage** represents bleeding of any part of the body, but the image above is an example of a brain hemorrhage. As you can see in *Figure 69* the white in the brain is blood and this is much more extensive than the previous small hemorrhage in *Figure 68*. The CSF is supposed to be able to circulate from the brain to the spine, but the blood is going into the ventricles and blocking them from receiving the CSF. There is mass effect upon the brain and the mid-line is shifting. Remember the brain must be symmetrical!

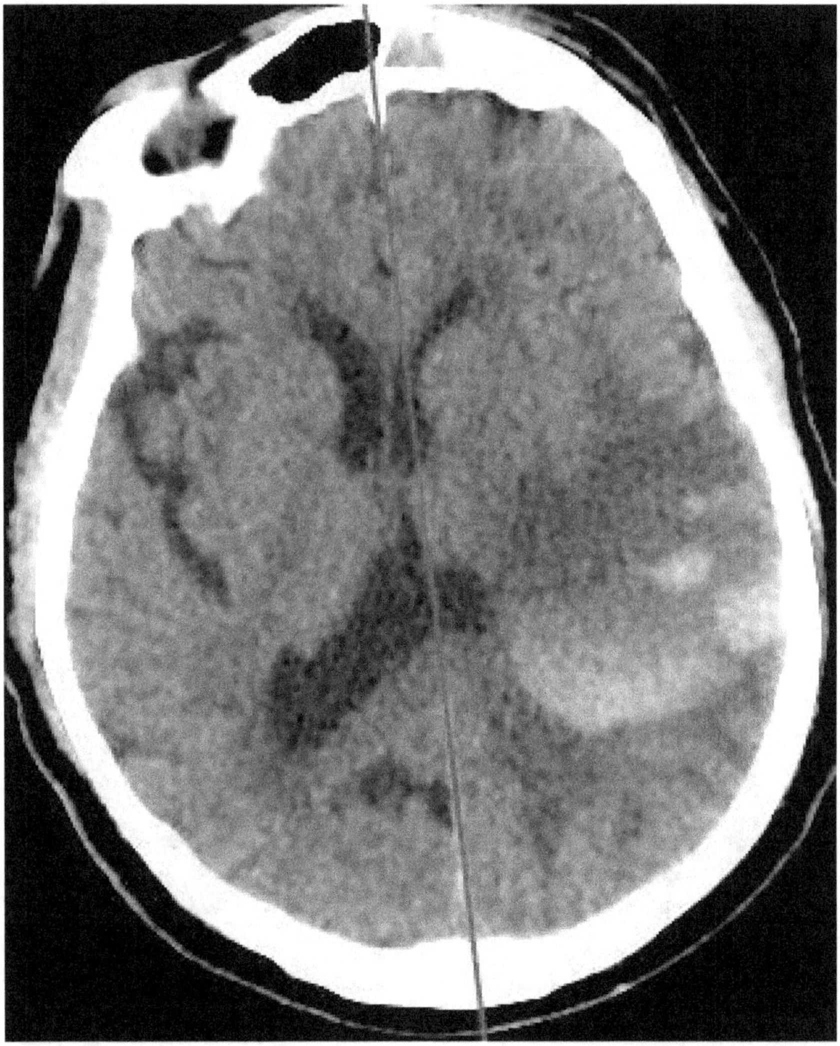

Figure 70. The vertical line drawn from anterior to posterior lies along the falx that separates the two cerebral hemispheres. The large left sided brain hemorrhage has caused the brain to shift towards the right and is no longer symmetric. Also notice enlargement of the right ventricle and compression of the left ventricle.

Midline shift means that one side of the brain moves over to the other side of the line that is drawn in *Figure 70*. The hemorrhage on the left side is causing the left brain to swell and moves some of the left brain over so it is no longer symmetric.

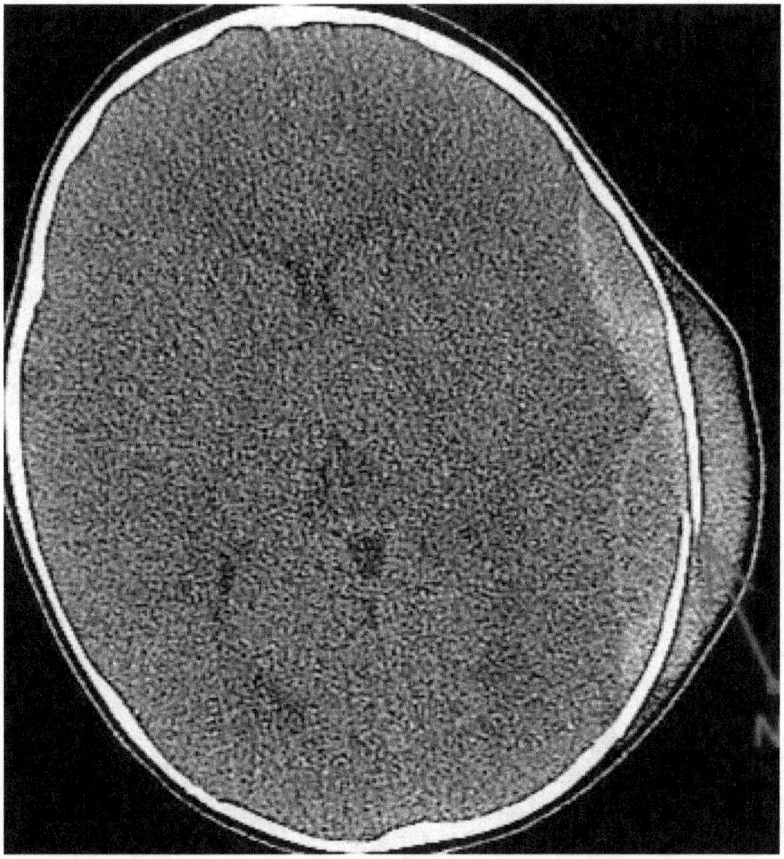

Figure 71. An axial CT showing blood on the inside of the brain associated with a skull fracture as well as blood causing a bump on the left scalp.

A **hematoma** is a blood clot that can be anywhere in or on the body. In *Figure 71*, the patient has a hematoma on the outside and inside of their brain due to an injury. The skull is the bright white line that wraps around the brain and there is a little fracture as indicated by the red arrow. As you can see, there is a large bump protruding out of the skull in the lighter grey, representing the hematoma. But there is also some lighter grey on the inside! Blood inside is the brain is not good! The brain should be symmetric but there is mass effect due to blood pushing the brain to the right which can cause a lot of internal brain problems.

Dealing with Brain Tumors

Ah, brain tumors - the unwelcome guests in our heads that nobody ever invited to the party. Let's put on our thinking caps (pun intended) as we dive into the world of dealing with brain tumors.

First things first, let's talk about what exactly a brain tumor is. In simple terms, it's like having a tiny squatter setting up camp in your brain without your permission. These pesky little growths can cause all sorts of trouble, from headaches to vision problems, and even changes in personality.

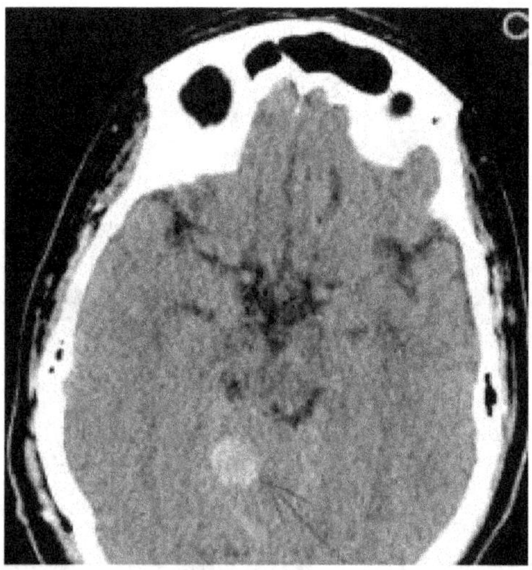

Figure 72. Not everything that is bright in the brain is blood. The arrow points to a small mass in the posterior right brain/ cerebellum.

Figure 72 is an example of a tumor as a round mass that is not a super bright white and is closer to a grey. This is the way you can tell the difference between a hemorrhage and a tumor because a hemorrhage is much brighter while a tumor is faintly bright. We cannot tell if it is a primary meaning the tumor is in its original starting place or a metastasis that has spread from a different part of the body.

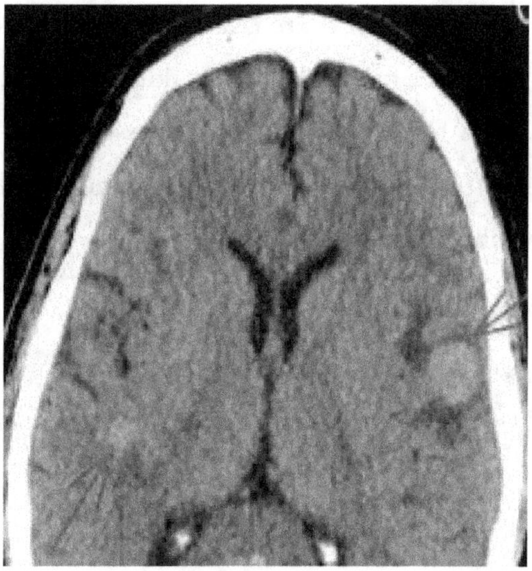

Figure 73. Axial noncontrast CT of the brain showing small round masses on either side of the brain.

In *Figure 73*, there are two tumors, which the arrows are pointing to, so we know this is most likely metastatic, meaning the cancer has spread from one area to these two places.

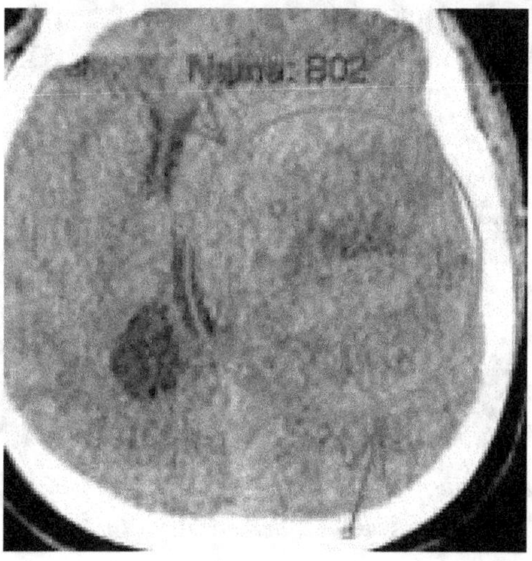

Figure 74. The circle shows a brain mass that causes swelling of the left aspect of the brain and midline shift. Notice the right ventricle posteriorly is enlarged due to obstruction of flow of CSF.

As you can see in *Figure 74* there is a mass circled in the left brain that is compressing the rest of the brain! The skull is almost like a container so there is no space for the right side of the brain to be pushed into. This causes mass effect, midline shift and dilatation of the ventricles, the darker grey parts in the brain containing CSF, so there is decrease flow of the CSF.

The good news is that not all brain tumors are malignant. The one below is typical of what is called a **meningioma**. This is seen along the surface of the skull and has calcifications which is the bright white - like the adjacent skull.

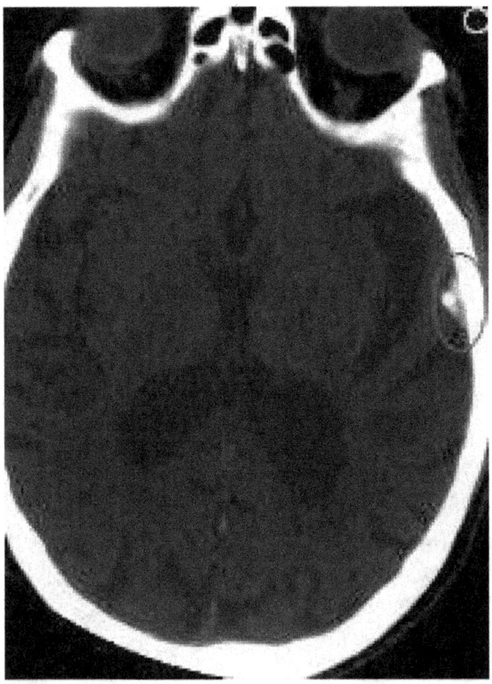

Figure 75. A small, calcified mass along the left skull inner aspect represents a meningioma, a benign brain tumor.

The mass in the right front of the brain circled, as shown in *Figure 75*, could be any type of tumor. This was in a 16-year-old.

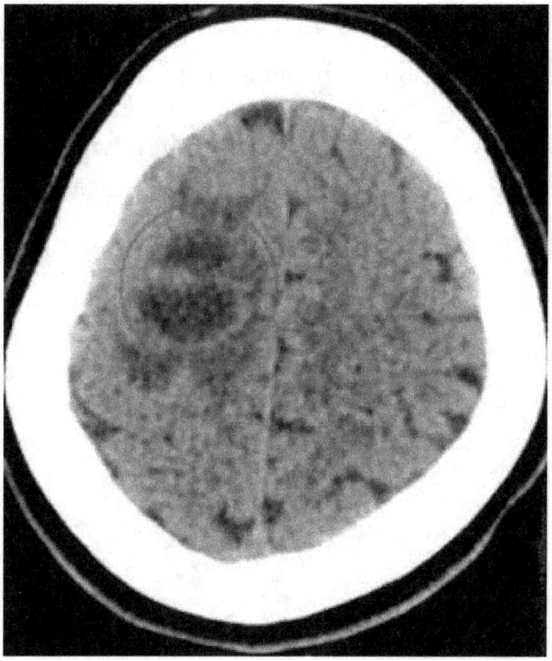

Figure 75. Circled is a round mass with central low density that is similar to the density of CSF.

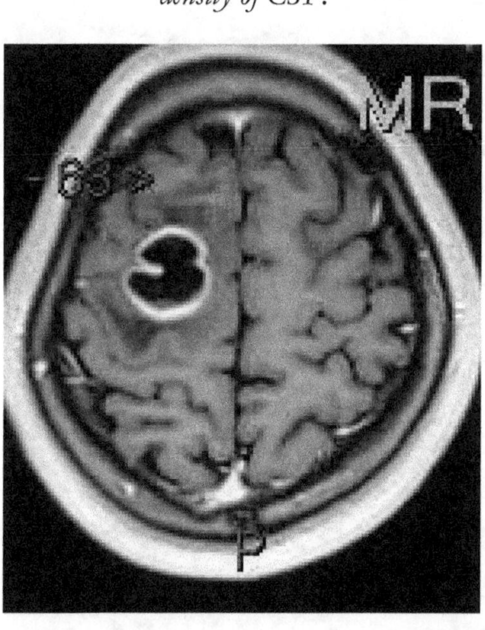

Figure 76. Post contrast MRI shows the right brain mass to be enhancing around the periphery and the central component is non-enhancing because it contains pus.

On the MR the lesion is enhancing around the edge and inside is cystic, and this turned out to be an abscess.

Now, you may be wondering how exactly we deal with these brain tumors once we've spotted them on a CT scan. Well, the good news is that there are a variety of treatment options available, ranging from surgery to radiation therapy. It's like playing a game of whack-a-mole, except instead of moles, we're dealing with tiny tumors in our brains. And trust me, the doctors are much better at this game than we are at the arcade.

CHAPTER 5
MUSCULOSKELETAL IMAGING AND DISEASES

EXAMINING BONES AND JOINTS

In this chapter, we'll be delving into the fascinating realm of bones and joints, examining how they work together to keep us moving and grooving.

First up, let's talk about bones. These hard, calcium-rich structures form the framework of our bodies, providing support and protection for our vital organs. Without bones, we'd be nothing more than a squishy blob of flesh flopping around aimlessly – not a pretty sight.

Now, onto joints – the hinges that allow our bones to move in harmony. From the ball-and-socket joint of the hip to the hinge joint of the knee, these cleverly designed connections enable us to bend, twist, and strut our stuff on the dance floor. Just imagine trying to break it down on the dance floor without your trusty joints – you'd be as stiff as a board!

SPORTS INJURIES

When it comes to examining bones and joints using CT scans, radiologists have a keen eye for detail. They can spot fractures, dislocations, and other issues that may be causing you pain or discomfort. Sports injuries can be a teen's worst nightmare, especially when it means missing out on all the action on the field. Just imagine having to sit on the sidelines while your friends are out there scoring goals or hitting home runs. It's enough to make anyone cringe in horror!

The basic Xray may seem normal, but there is still a possibility of significant injury to the soft tissues adjacent to the bones that cannot be seen by Xrays alone; Xrays can only see the calcification of the bones. So specialized imaging such as MRI is needed to see structural abnormalities that one cannot otherwise evaluate. For example, ligaments, short bands of tough, flexible, fibrous, connective tissue that connect two bones or cartilages or hold together a joint, can be seen on MRI but are not visible on Xrays.

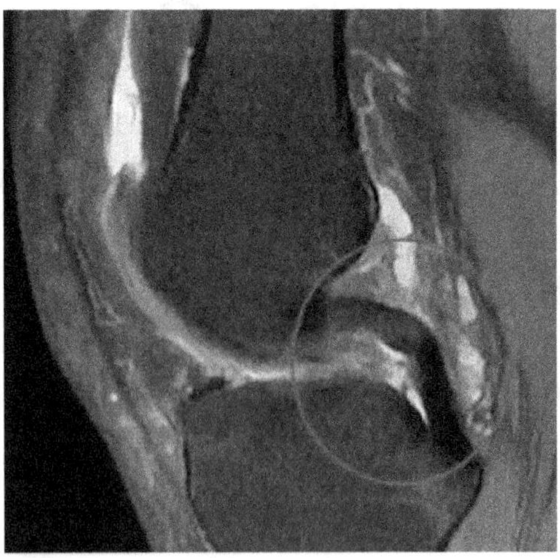

Figure 77. Sagittal MRI shows a normal appearance of tendons and ligaments with a black homogenous appearance as in this case of a normal posterior cruciate ligament.

Figure 77 is an example of a normal **black posterior cruciate ligament- PCL**. This blackness, circled, is how the **anterior cruciate ligament** (ACL) should normally look when it is not torn. The PCL and ACL are on different sides of the knee as one is posterior and the other is anterior, but their appearance should be the same on an MRI scan.

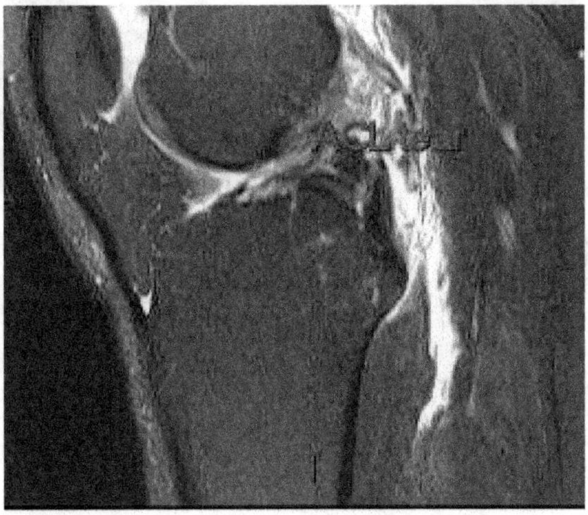

Figure 78. Notice that this ligament called the anterior cruciate ligament that crosses the knee is ill defined and grey compared to the PCL which lies behind it. This is indicative of an ACL tear.

In *Figure 78* the ACL is fuzzy, ill-defined, and too wide meaning it is torn! Normal ligaments are a thinner line and are darker. Many athletes experience ACL tears typically where jumping, pivoting, and abrupt change in direction while running occur. This can cause pain and swelling, but can be rehabilitated with surgery and physical therapy.

When an Xray cannot find a subtle fracture and the severity of the pain makes the patient or doctor think there is something more going on, then more specialized imaging such as CT or MRI may be needed. For example, where is the fracture in *Figure 79*? Not visible!

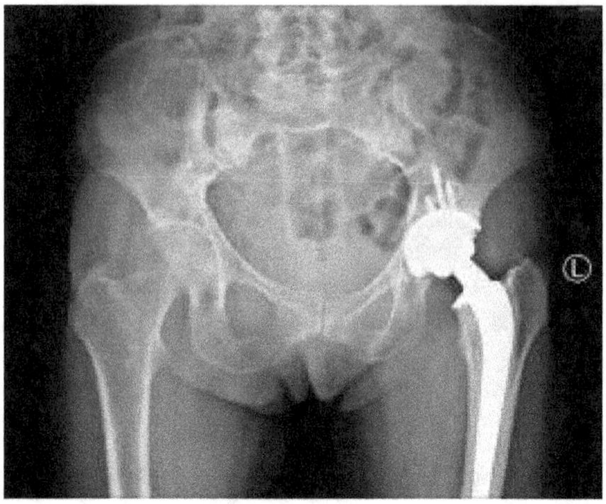

Figure 79. A plain Xray of the pelvis shows a left hip replacement. A fracture line cannot be definitively seen in the right hip onto which the patient fell and where the patient has pain.

Even when the area of concern is circled, no one can confidently call a fracture on the Xray in *Figure 79*. This is when the superhero of MRI comes into action to save the day. So, if the doctor has a high suspicion for a fracture, they can order an MRI to figure out for sure if there is a fracture or not.

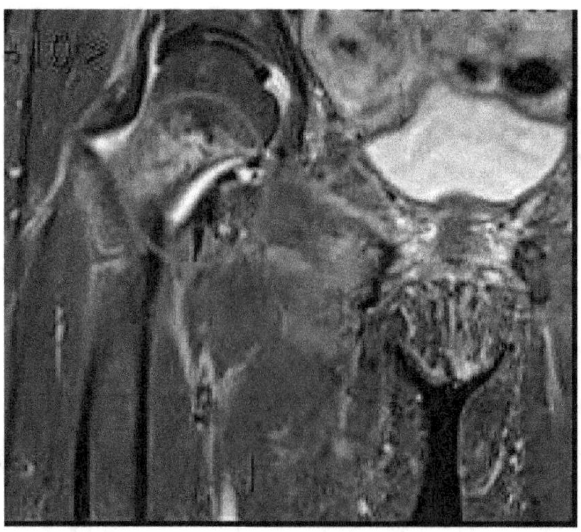

Figure 80. MRI STIR sequence that accentuates fluid has an area of edema that is circled in the right femoral neck.

On this sequence in Figure 80, where water shows up as bright as the bladder does, the big white blob in the picture, there is a bright signal in the right femur. This signals edema or bruising of the bone, therefore, the radiologist knows to look more carefully in this region. In another sequence (*Figure 81*) the line of the fracture in the right femur can easily be seen.

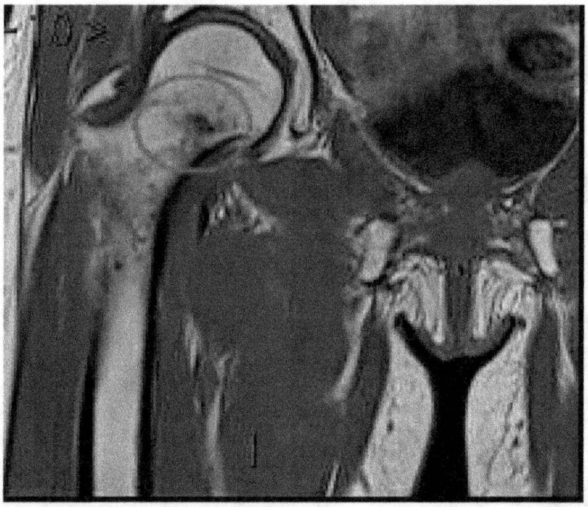

Figure 81. A different MRI sequence which is better for anatomy shows a linear area of black in the region of the right femoral neck demonstrating a fracture line.

Now the patient can be appropriately treated and know the diagnosis instead of walking on that hip and causing more injury.

ARTHRITIS: NOT JUST FOR GRANDMA

You may think arthritis is just something that old people get but arthritis can affect people of all ages, including kids. That's right, arthritis doesn't discriminate based on age - it can sneak up on anyone, even the hippest and happening adolescents. This is why it is important to stay active and healthy!

Now, before you start panicking and picturing yourself hobbling around with a cane at the ripe old age of 16, let's break it down a bit. Arthritis is basically inflammation in your joints, which can cause pain, stiffness, and swelling. It's like your body's way of reminding you to take it easy and not overdo it at the skate park or during that intense game of basketball.

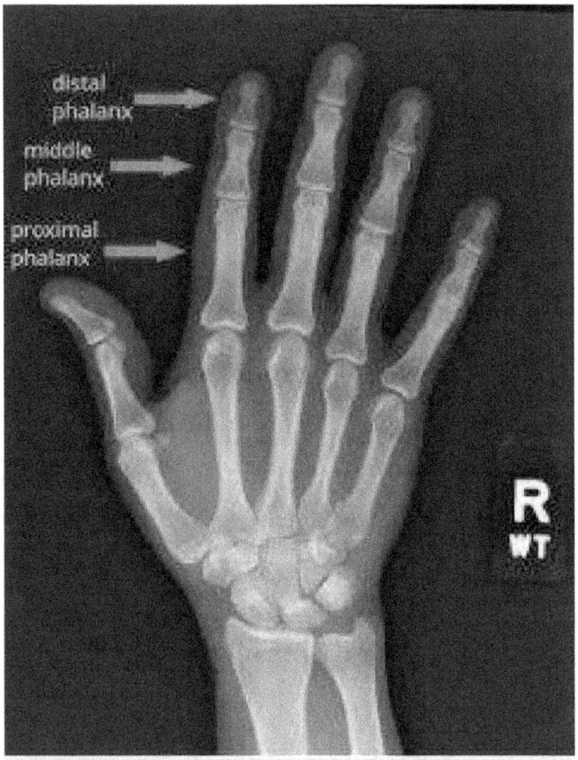

Figure 82. Plain Xray of the right hand demonstrating a normal appearance to the digits of the hand and their labels. Notice the spaces between the joints are well maintained.

A normal hand has the distal phalanx, middle phalanx, and proximal phalanx as the three bones that make up each finger. In between each phalanx, there is a bit of space (a joint space), which allows people to move their fingers freely. When there is minimal space in those areas, that is a sign of arthritis.

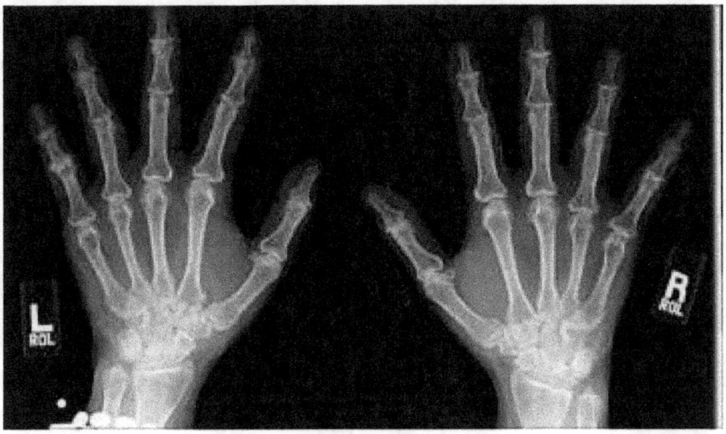

Figure 83. Plain Xray of both hands with narrowing of the joint spaces in this patient with quite advanced osteoarthritis.

Demonstrated in the image above is the classic appearance of osteoarthritis because as you can see there is very little space between each portion of each finger – the phalangeal bone. It almost seems clustered together.

One of the earliest signs of osteoarthritis is narrowing at the bottom of the thumb called the carpometacarpal joint.

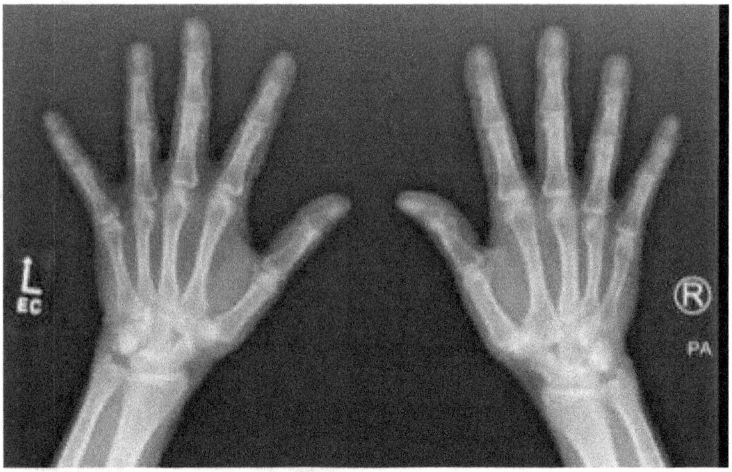

Figure 84. Early signs of osteoarthritis are mild narrowing of the thumb carpometacarpal joint.

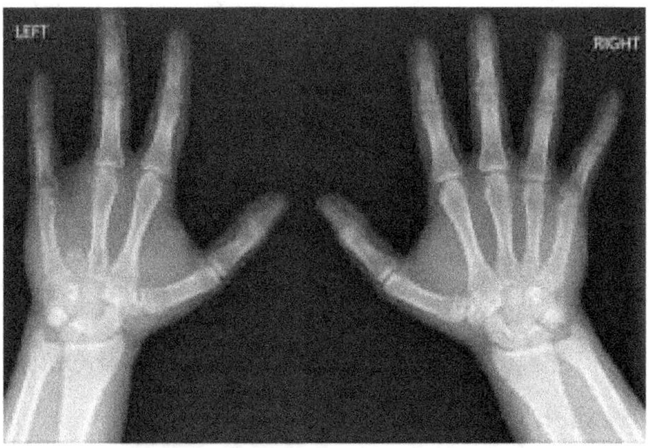

Figure 85. This plain Xray shows circled the normal appearance of the thumb carpometacarpal joints on each side as a comparison.

Did you notice something about the left hand- yes, the fourth or ring finger has been amputated (cut off)?

Like the hands, the normal knees have the bones with space in between them. The femur is the top bone which goes all the way up to the hip while the bottom bones are the tibia (the bigger one) and the fibula. The round circle just above the space, called the knee joint space, is the patella or the knee cap.

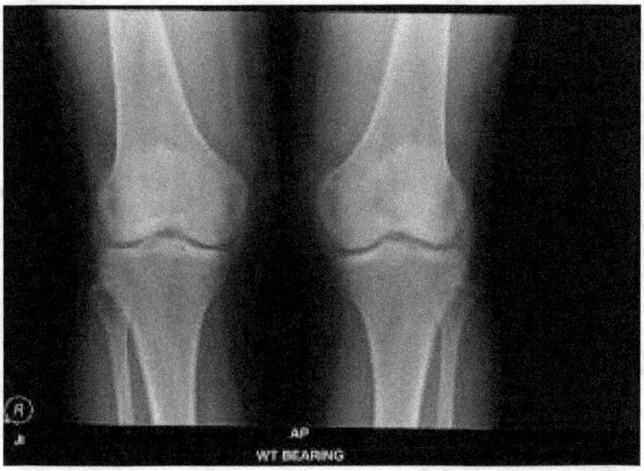

Figure 86. Plain frontal Xray of the knees showing normal joint spaces and positioning.

Osteoarthritis is the most common type of arthritis (inflammation of the joints) that occurs with wear and tear when a joint space is narrowed, typically associated with osteophytes or small spur like pointy projections.

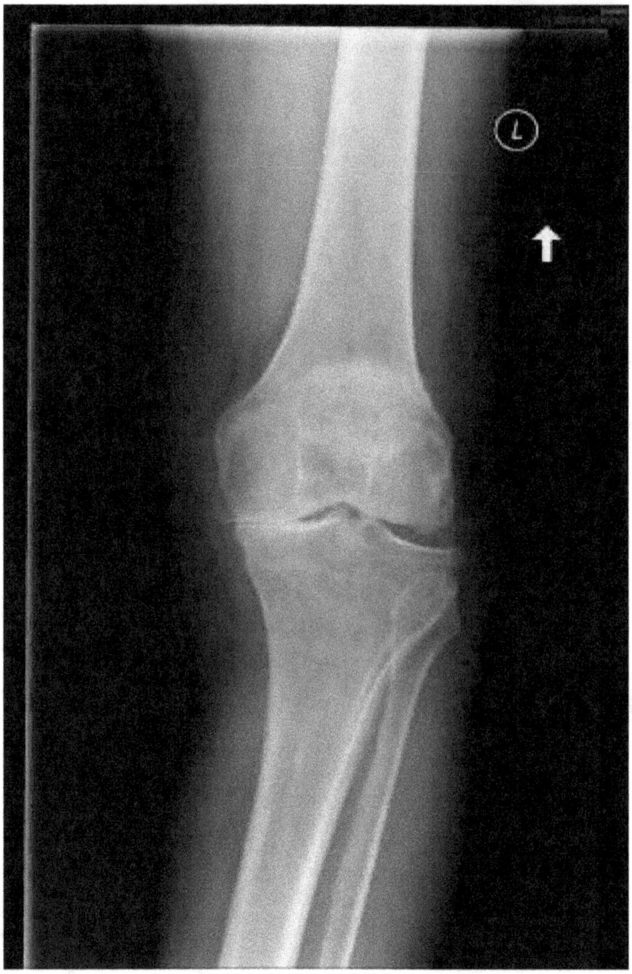

Figure 87. Plain Xray showing severe narrowing of the knee joint along the medial aspect with complete loss of joint space.

The fibula is the little bone of the calf that lies along the lateral aspect of the leg, so we can see that the medial cushion at the ends of bones (the cartilage) has worn down and now the two bones are touching each other. The image above is an example of osteoarthritis of the medial (inner side) of the left knee. Compared to *Figure 86*, the space is more cramped, causing pain and decreased mobility.

But fear not, my young friends! Just because arthritis can happen to us doesn't mean we're doomed to a life of early bird specials and rocking chairs. With proper care, exercise, and maybe a little less time spent on our phones, we can keep arthritis at bay and continue living our best, pain-free lives.

BONE CANCER.

Next let's take a look at something that eats away at the bone itself. Take a second to compare the right and left femur which are the hip bones on this X-ray. The right femur has a mottled appearance because it is being eaten up by a tumor. This is the most common bone cancer, **osteosarcoma**. It is vital that cancer is caught in time, so it does not spread through the blood to the lungs, liver, and rest of the body. Right now, the osteosarcoma is only in the bone, so it can be treated before it gets a chance to spread to the rest of the body and become lethal.

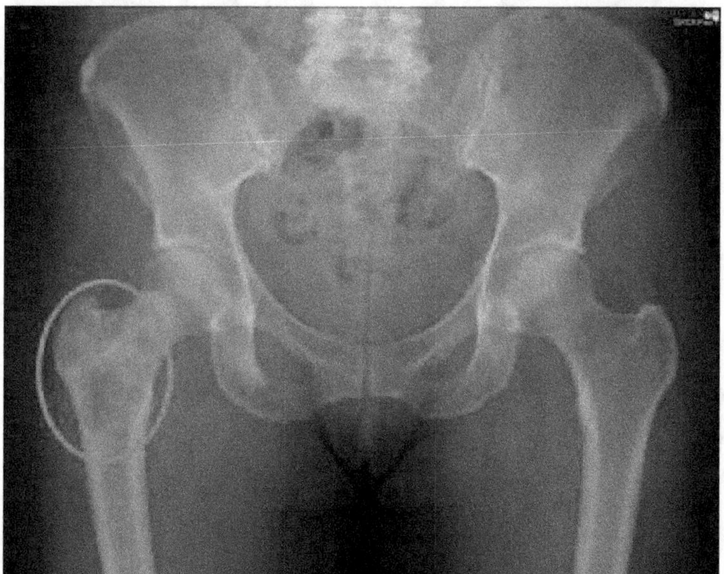

Figure 88. Plain Xray of the pelvis shows an area of heterogenous appearance to the right proximal femur.

This is the same patient with the osteosarcoma except now it is shown on a CT scan. The osteosarcoma appears to have a brighter appearance because the tumor produces bone compared to the left femur and it is almost as if there are bubbles present within the bone. Not good!

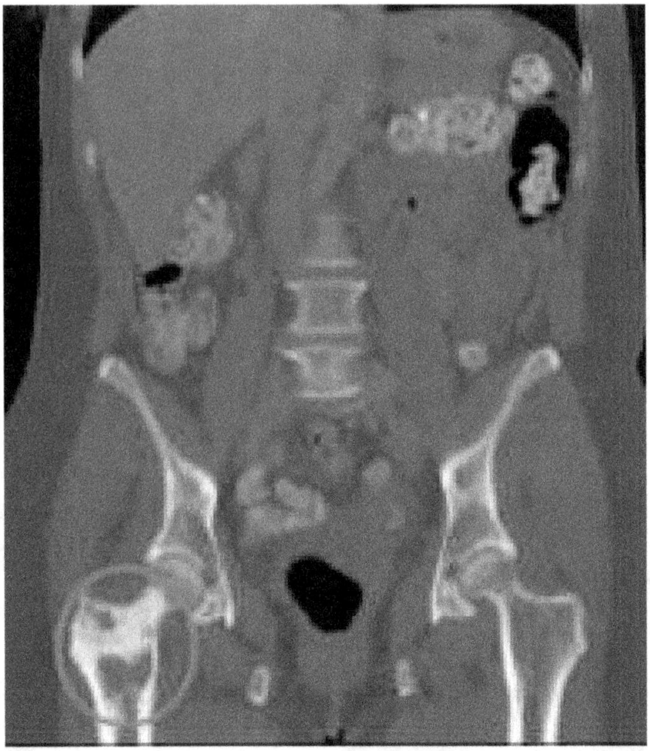

Figure 89. Coronal CT shows the heterogenous mottled area of the right proximal femur circled.

In conclusion, bones and joints are like the dynamic duo of the human body, working together to keep us upright and mobile. Through the lens of radiology, we can explore these intricate structures in stunning detail, gaining a deeper understanding of how they function and what happens when things go awry.

CHAPTER 6

RADIOLOGY PROCEDURES

CT GUIDED DRAINAGE OF ABSCESS DUE TO APPENDICITIS.

So, we have gone through many of the complications that can happen to your body, but what we have not discussed is how radiologists can fix these problems to help the patient feel better. Radiologists actually have to interact with patients!

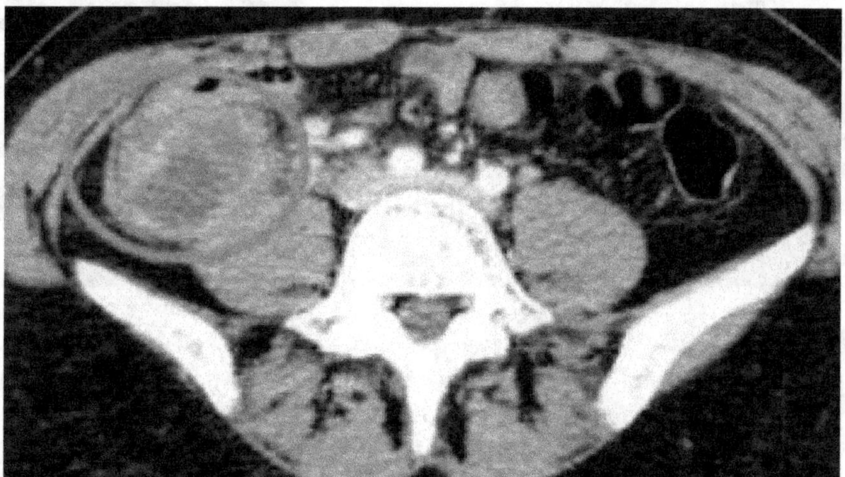

Figure 90. Axial CT through the pelvis shows an abscess in the right abdomen that was the result of an episode of appendicitis.

As you know now, the appendix is a small blind-ending tube that is attached to the end of the cecum and can become inflamed resulting in appendicitis. But what can happen if the appendix bursts from appendicitis? *Figure 90* is an example of a possible outcome where the pus from the appendix can form an abscess (a ball of pus). The radiologist needs to do a procedure so that the abscess does not get bigger any larger, because then it could spread to the bloodstream which would cause sepsis, a fatal infection. One way an abscess can be treated without surgery is by the radiologist placing a drain under CT guidance.

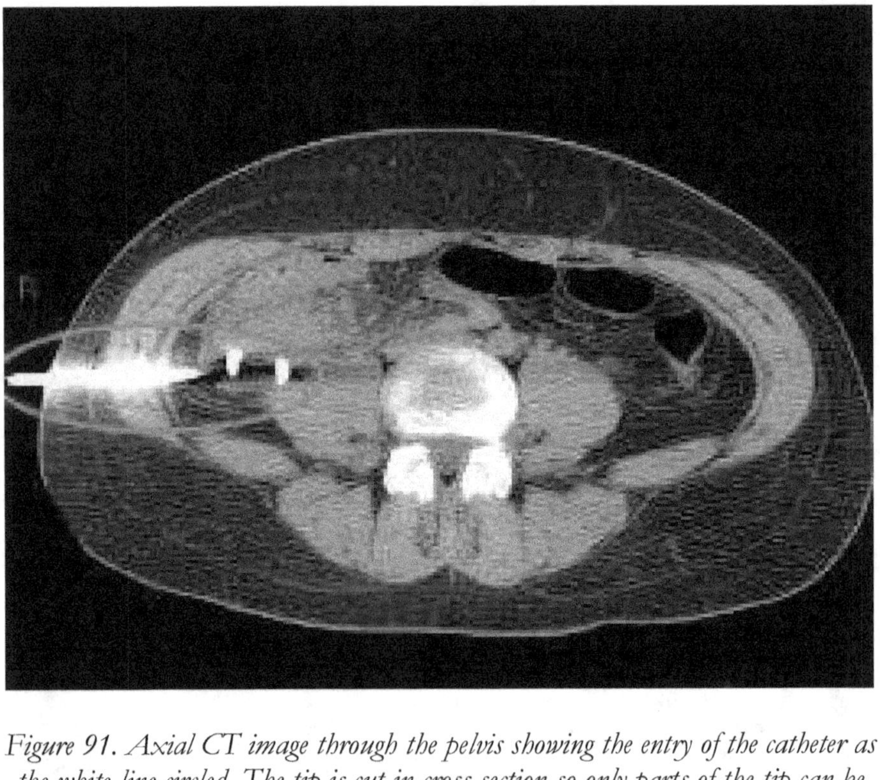

Figure 91. Axial CT image through the pelvis showing the entry of the catheter as the white line circled. The tip is cut in cross section so only parts of the tip can be seen on this image, but it is coiled hence the name pigtail catheter.

The horizontal white line with metal artifact is the drain.

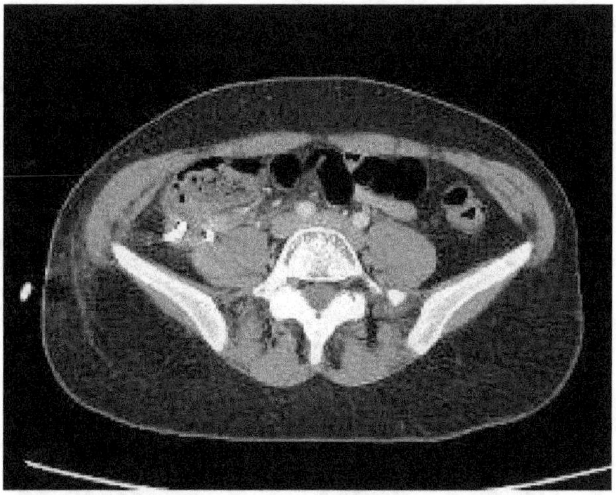

Figure 92. Axial CT of the pelvis demonstrates the pigtail catheter tip in the right pelvis with resolution of the abscess. Anterior to the catheter is the normal right colon with the mottled appearance being feces.

One week later after a drain is inserted into the abscess, the abscess is smaller and the patient can then go to surgery to remove the appendix.

Next let's take a look at this liver (*Figure 93*)- there are some grey splotches in the liver representing an abscess that is circled. Like with the appendiceal abscess, the radiologist is able to insert a drain into the liver abscess to let the pus exit the body and treat the patient.

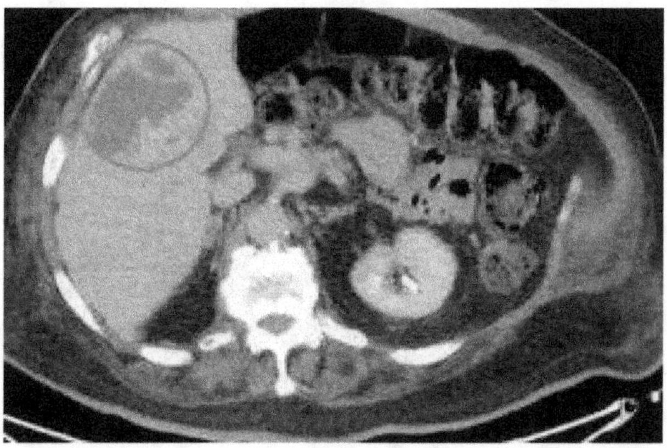

Figure 93. Axial CT of the abdomen shows a liver abscess within the circle.

As a result of using the drain, the patient does not have to go to surgery. In the image below, the white line is called a **pigtail catheter** because of the shape of the tip which curves like a pig's tail to keep itself inside the abscess, so it is locked in place. Can you find the abscess anymore? No, because it's been drained out! Now the catheter can be removed, and the patient does not need surgery.

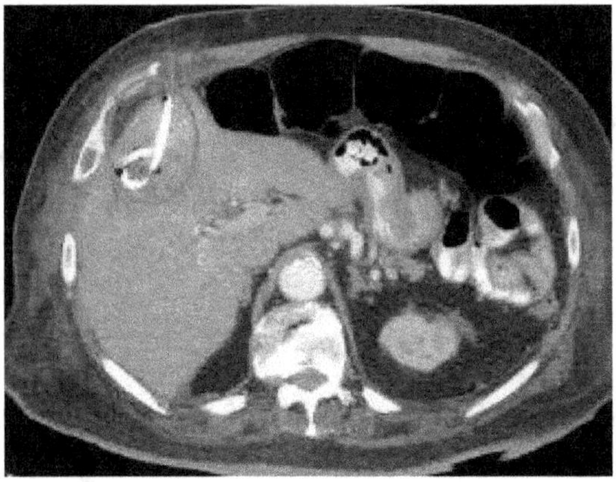

Figure 94. Axial CT of the abdomen shows entry of a pigtail catheter from the anterior right abdomen into the liver abscess. Notice the coiling of the tip – the reason for its name pigtail.

Next let's look at a lung biopsy. The lungs do not look normal in this image!

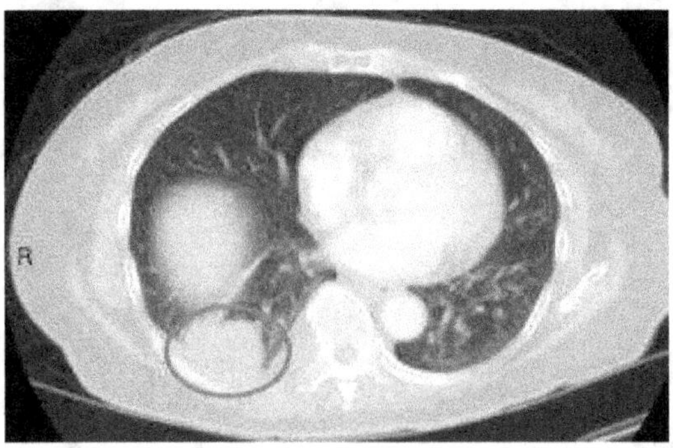

Figure 95. Axial CT of the lung bases with lung windows demonstrates a large mass at the right lung base.

In the bottom right lung, there is a large mass that is touching the ribs. You might be wondering, what about that white blob in the lung in front of the mass that is circled (*Figure 95*)? That is a part of the body- the liver. It just looks odd because this is just a slice of the body, and this is an artifact called "volume averaging".

The patient must be placed on their tummy so that the lung mass can be accessed by the needle in the safest way. Multiple images during the placement of the needle are taken to guide the needle into the appropriate position before taking samples, and to avoid hitting the liver which lies right next to the mass. The procedure done here is called a **<u>CT guided right lung mass biopsy</u>** where the radiologist takes a few tiny samples to look under the microscope to figure out whether the mass is cancer and its specific type or whether it is benign and can be watched.

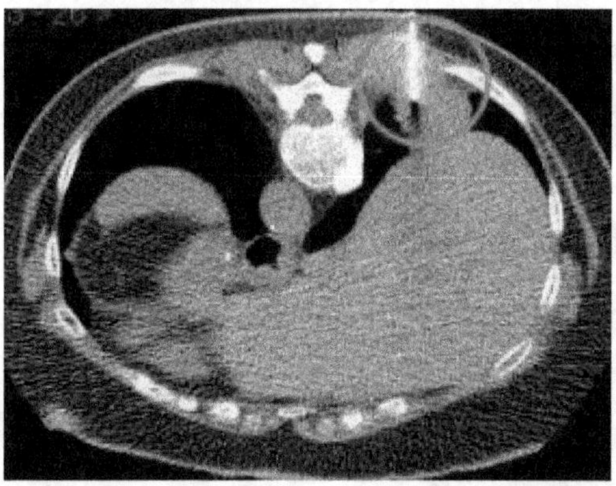

Figure 96. The patient was placed prone to provide easy access through the back to the lung mass to decrease potential injury to the adjacent organs.

What happens if one of the kidneys has been removed and the remaining kidney develops a mass such as in *Figure 97*? In this case the left kidney has already been removed due to cancer. A small right renal mass that has developed can be ablated- killed with either heat, microwave or freezing therapy called cryoablation- to avoid surgery and removal of the remaining kidney.

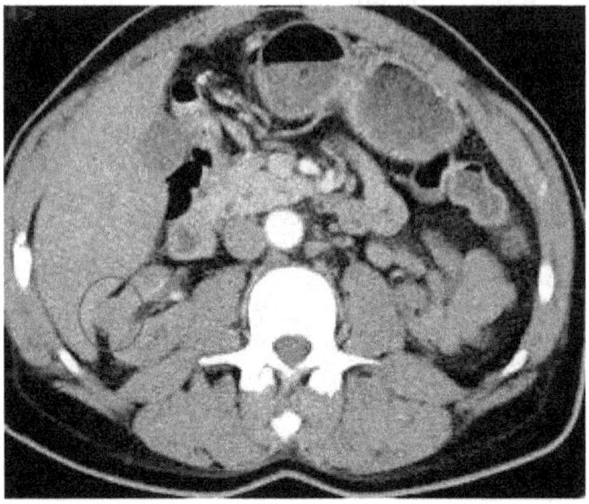

Figure 97. Axial CT of the liver demonstrates a small round mass in the mid right kidney as circled.

Like the lung mass, the radiologist can put in a needle under CT guidance with the patient turned on their tummy. Then the radiologist can biopsy the mass and at the same time can instill heat or cooling through the special ablation/biopsy needle to kill the cells that make up the mass. This avoids the patient going to surgery and saves them having to remove the only kidney they have.

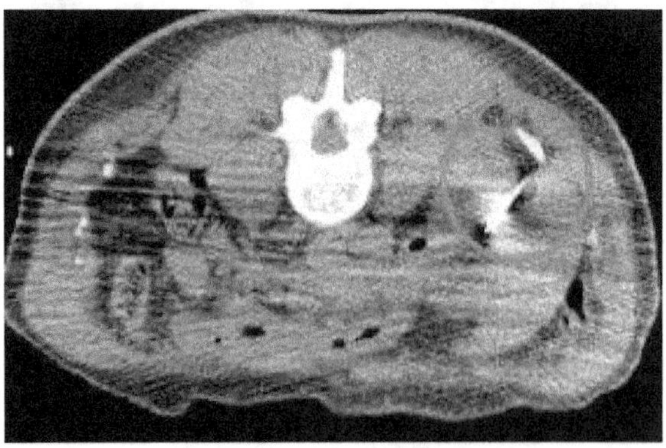

Figure 98. Axial CT of the abdomen with the patient prone (lying on the tummy) to provide a safer access to biopsy the right renal mass.

The next case is a pelvic peritoneal nodule, separate from the organs. Peritoneal means it's within the abdomen that surrounds the bowel, like a lining or a bedsheet. Since the mass is enhancing or lighting up with contrast, the mass does not represent a cyst, meaning that it cannot be characterized as benign on imaging. Therefore a biopsy is needed for further evaluation.

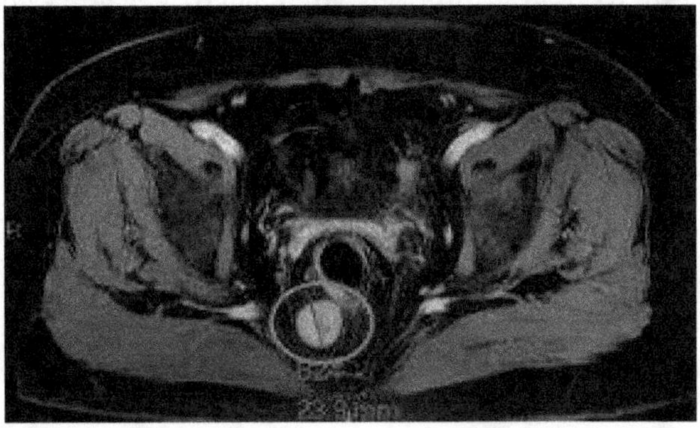

Figure 99. Axial MRI of the pelvis shows a round enhancing mass in the posterior pelvis as circled.

They biopsied this mass in the same way as they did the lung and liver masses and found out that it was cancer!

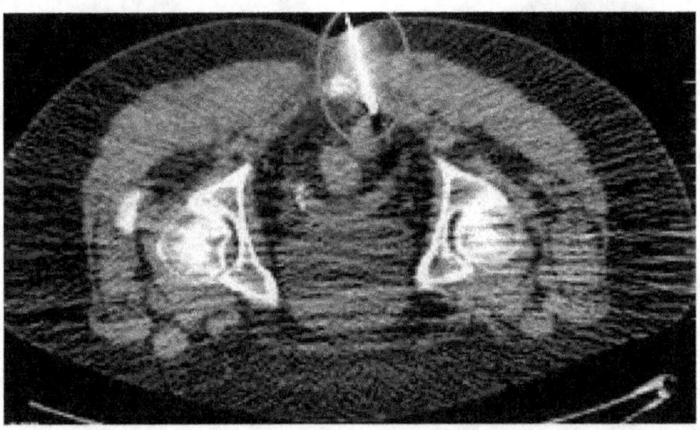

Figure 100. The patient is placed prone to provide safe access to biopsy the mass. The radiologist has to try to go as medial and inferiorly as possible next to the sacrum and coccyx- the lower most back bones that we sit on so that the sciatic nerve is avoided.

These examples, previously mentioned, have been of procedures done under CT guidance and these are sometimes but not necessarily performed by an interventional radiologist. The more complex interventional radiology procedures can involve injecting dye through the groin (through the common femoral artery) via long catheters that can be manipulated under X-ray/fluoroscopic guidance to parts of the brain and body to treat conditions such as strokes and cancers without major surgery. This is beyond the scope of this book.

How crazy is it that radiologists can be like surgeons in how they do procedures, just they don't cut open the patient? There are so many specialties available!

CHAPTER 7
THE ROLE OF ARTIFICIAL INTELLIGENCE

ARTIFICIAL INTELLIGENCE (AI) HELPS...SOMETIMES

The rumor that "artificial intelligence will take over the field of radiology" should probably be taken with a pinch of salt. Artificial intelligence or AI has been available for decades in radiology and is only getting better but this is to the advantage of the radiologist. AI overall improves their daily activities. It can facilitate the triaging/prioritization of more urgent studies that require attention from a long list of studies. Additionally, AI can help make the radiologist aware of subtle findings, or areas that need a second look so the radiologist can check if the abnormality the AI service is picking up is a true finding or not. Radiologists are not threatened by AI, as they see the many studies AI gets wrong, of which a seasoned radiologist can easily decipher correctly. However, AI can be helpful because it gives an added pair of eyes to zone in on subtle abnormalities that may not be noticed otherwise.

Here are some examples:

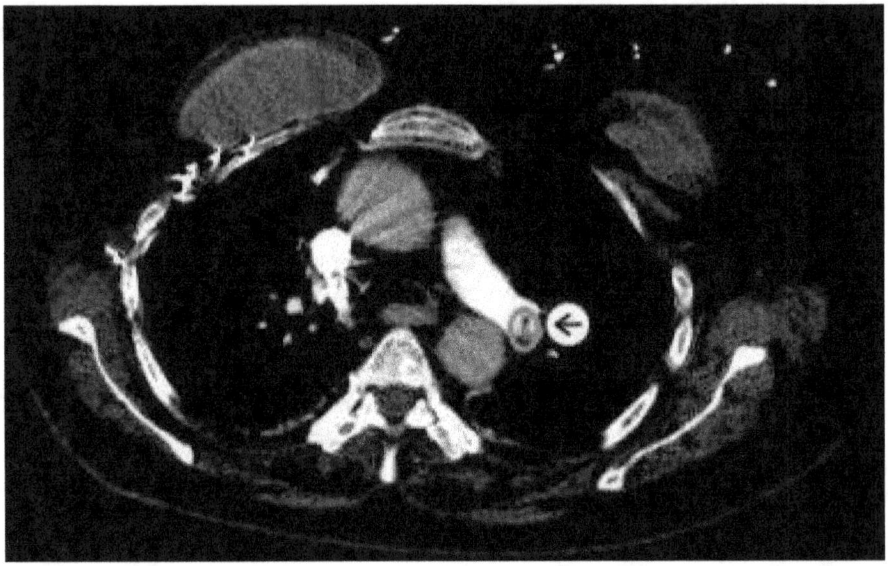

Figure 101. Axial CT of the chest with mediastinal windows demonstrating a filling defect as circled in the left pulmonary artery that the AI is pointing an arrow toward.

AI points to an area that it thinks is a pulmonary embolism (remember that is a blood clot in the artery of the lung) in the left pulmonary artery. When carefully examining this area, it can be seen just to be the bifurcation (splitting) of the left pulmonary artery causing an artifact (*Figure 102*). The same level is depicted by the line drawn on the coronal images and no filling defect is seen to corroborate the AI finding. The green line is where we would expect to see a filling defect to show a sign of a pulmonary embolism (a blood clot stuck in the pulmonary artery), but there is none so this is a false positive for AI.

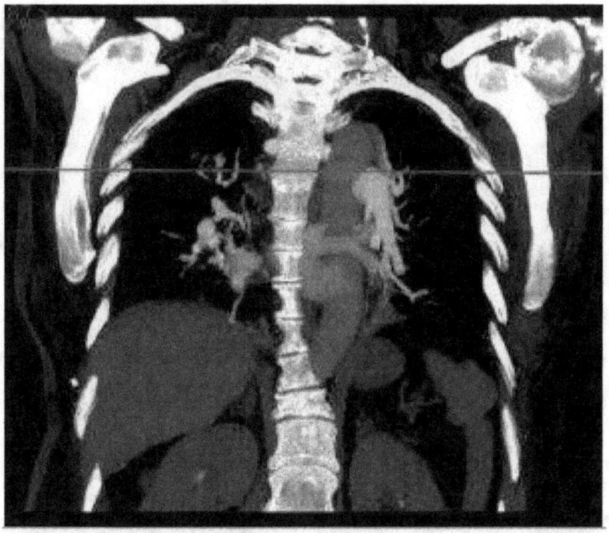

Figure 102. Coronal CT image with the horizontal line corresponding to the abnormality reported by AI application.

Here in *Figure 103*, the AI is pointing to the right-side pulmonary artery where there appears to be a big round filling defect, circled in the red. The AI is calling a pulmonary embolism, but in actuality, it is a large, abnormal lymph node. Again, this is a false positive.

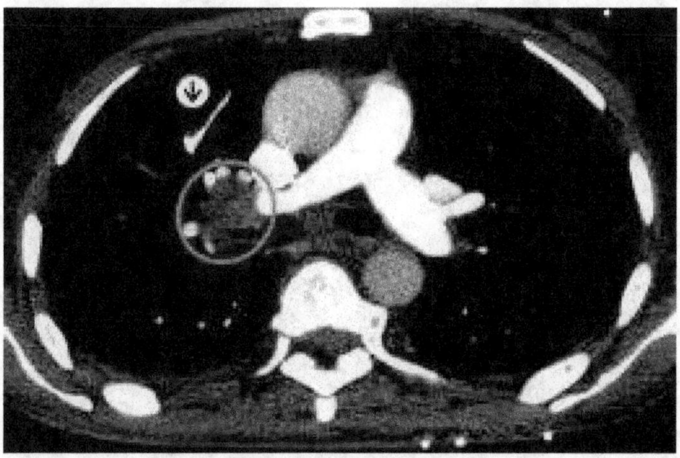

Figure 103. AI points to a filling defect in the region of the right pulmonary artery which turns out to be an enlarged lymph node and not a pulmonary embolism.

Another example is where the AI says no pulmonary embolism.

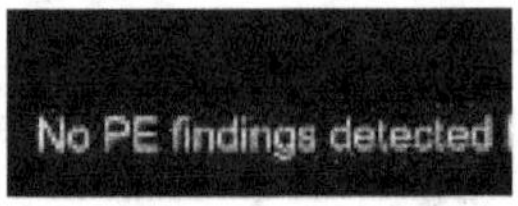

Figure 104. The notification that the AI application has finished processing the images and come to its conclusion when it is negative for pulmonary embolism.

But when examining the images carefully, a tiny filling defect is present in the left lower lobe pulmonary artery branch in the back and bottom of the lungs. The filling defect can be seen on the axial images and the coronal images as circled. This is a false negative for AI.

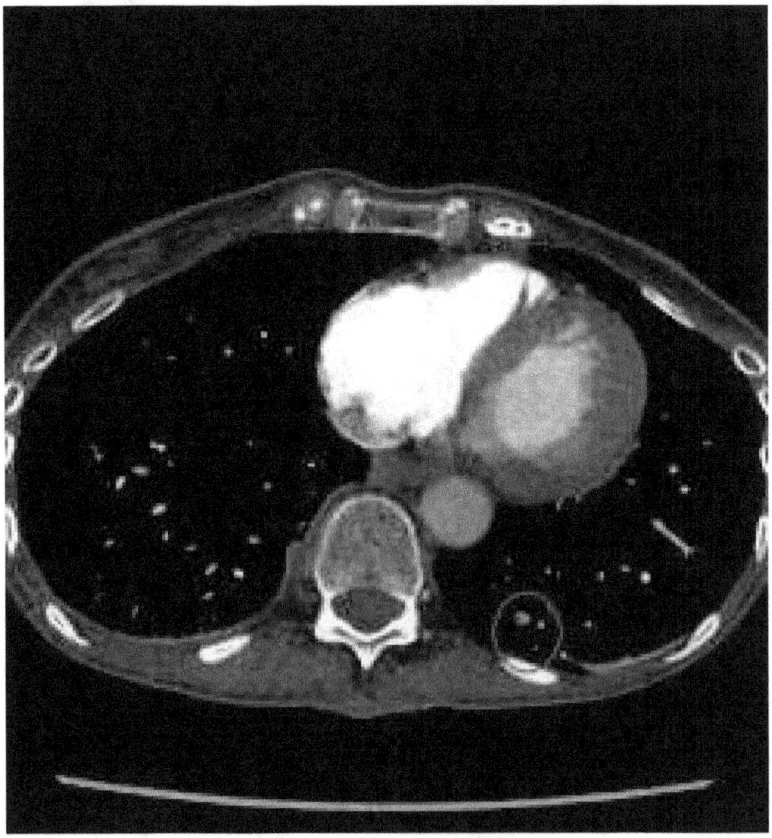

Figure 105. Axial close up of the left lower lobe pulmonary artery branches shows a tiny filling defect within the circled area.

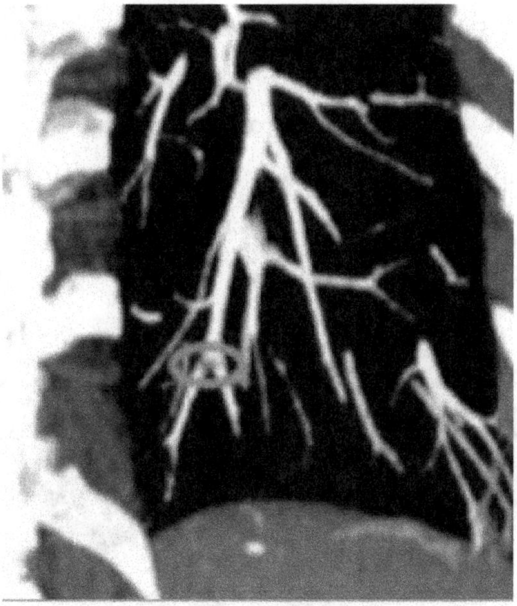

Figure 106. Coronal CT confirms a filling defect at the bifurcation (splitting) of the lower lobe branches of the left lower lobe pulmonary artery confirming a pulmonary embolism.

However, AI can often be helpful in finding tiny filling defects such as in this case below. AI shows an image so this alerts the radiologist to look carefully in this area.

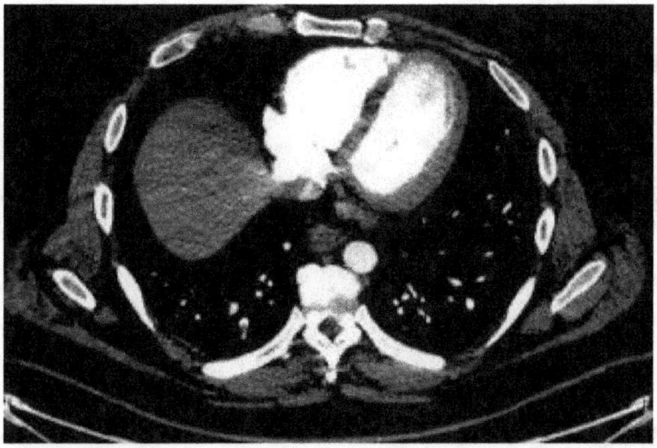

Figure 107. AI provides a notification that this image has a suspected pulmonary embolism.

A tiny filling defect can be seen in the right lower lobe pulmonary artery correlating to the finding pointed out by the AI, so the patient has a pulmonary embolism. This is a true positive and is an example of how AI can be helpful. If the pulmonary embolism gets too big, it can become lethal because it would block blood flow to the lungs, as a pulmonary embolism is blockage one or more arteries in the lungs by a blood clot.

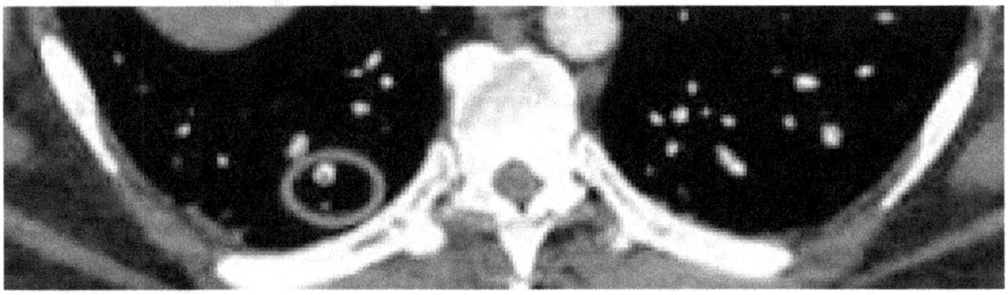

Figure 108. Circled is the small pulmonary artery branch containing a dot of grey that represents the tiny pulmonary embolism.

An emergency that we talked about earlier is free air in the abdomen which can indicate a bowel rupture. AI has so many applications but one such application can alert the radiologist to an area where it thinks there may be free air. Here is an example.

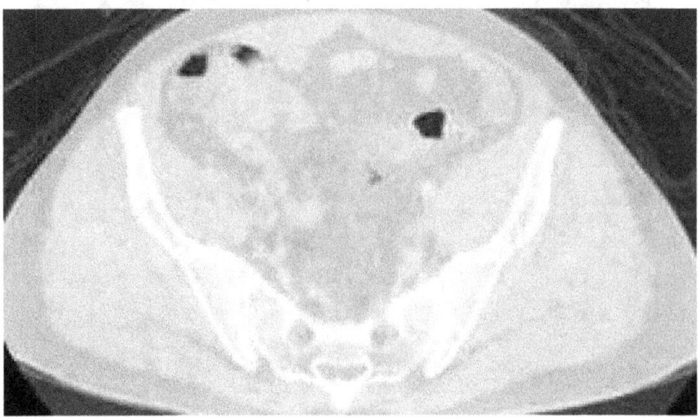

Figure 109. Axial CT of the pelvis highlighted by the AI application. The lung windows as provided accentuate free air.

The AI shows this image for the radiologist to pay special attention to. On careful review, the site of localized free intraperitoneal (inside the abdomen) air or a localized perforation from the sigmoid (the colon just above the rectum), where diverticulitis is the cause, is circled below.

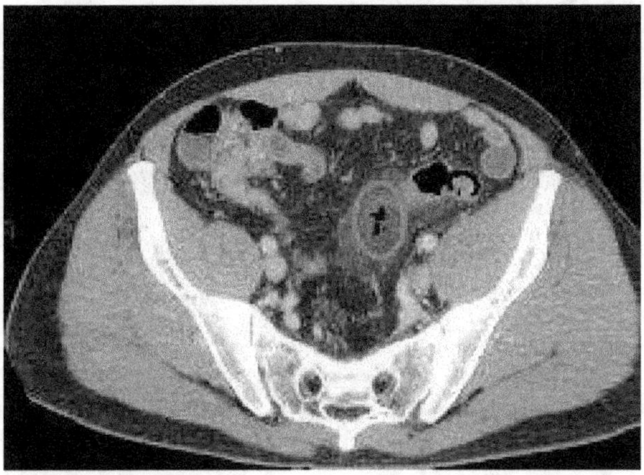

Figure 110. Concentrating on the image highlighted by the AI application one can find a small focus of free air that is circled above.

Sometimes AI can miss important findings.

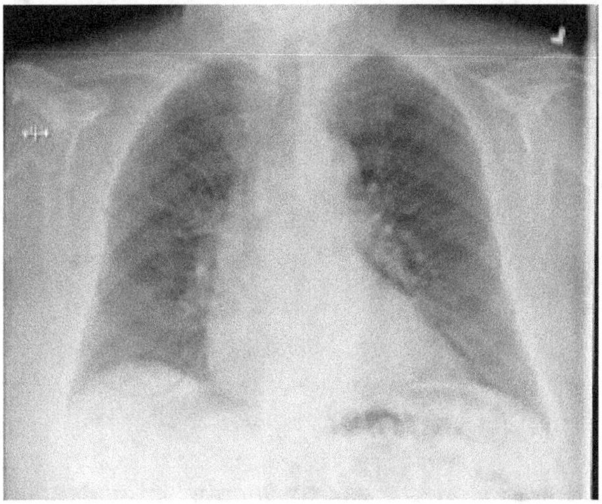

Figure 111. Plain frontal Xray of the chest. Notice the right lung base where the diaphragm is circled. There is lucency/grey amidst the white of the diaphragm that is circled.

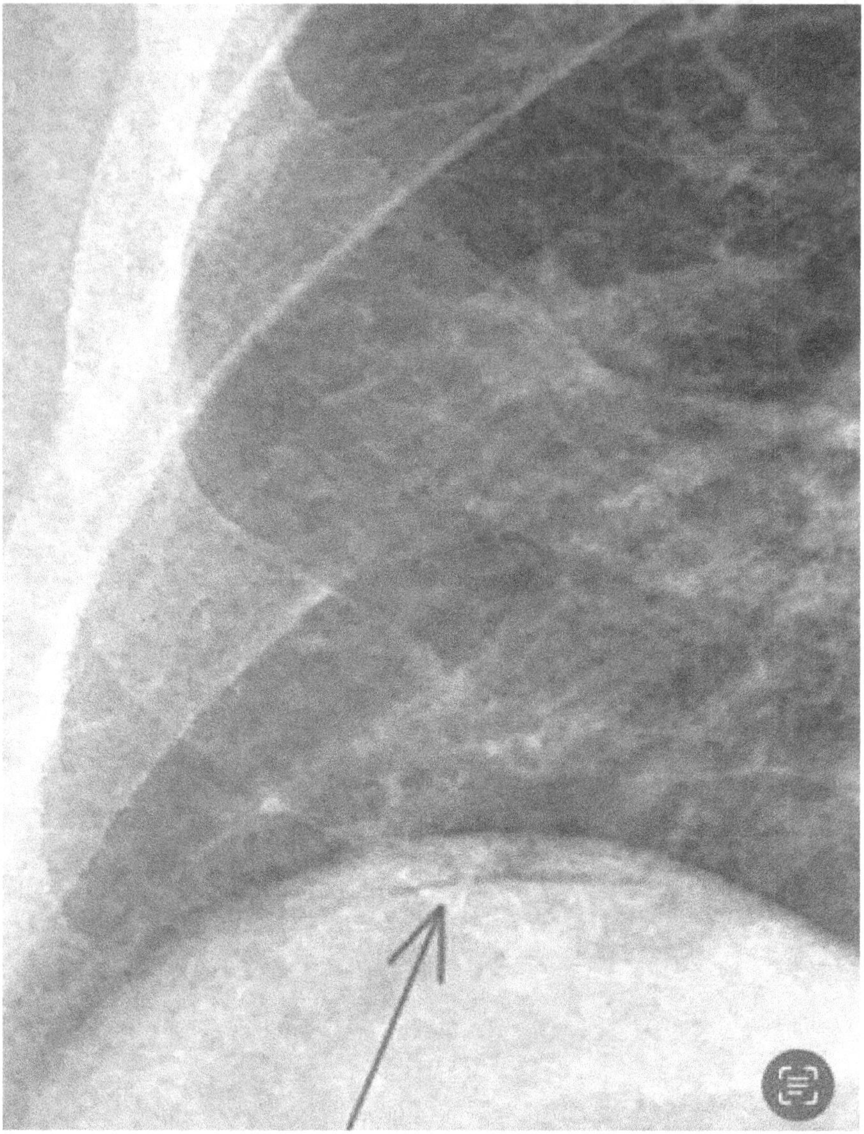

Figure 111b. Close up of the right hemidiaphragm demonstrates a small black curved area representing air beneath that hemidiaphragm so this is free air or pneumoperitoneum.

This patient had a chest Xray for a cough. Incidentally noted was a tiny sliver of lucency (circled) beneath the right hemidiaphragm. This raised concern for free intraperitoneal air, a finding that can denote bowel rupture. Thus, the patient had a CT for evaluation or confirmation. Small amounts of free intraperitoneal air were not called on by the AI for the patient below. Free air is best seen on lung windows.

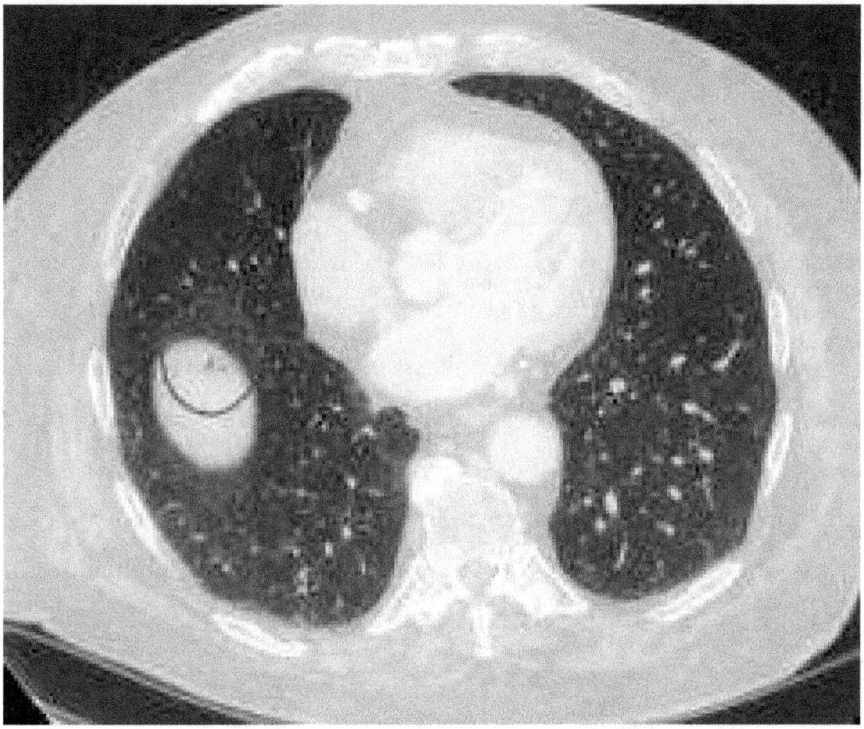

Figure 112. Axial CT image with lung windows demonstrates tiny dots of free air underneath the right hemidiaphragm corresponding to the air seen on chest x-ray.

In addition, the patient had pneumatosis which is air in the wall of the bowel. This can be seen when the bowel is infracting or dying, for example in *Figure 113*, so it's very important not to rely on a computer or AI as these are life and death situations. A trained radiologist is needed to decipher complex situations.

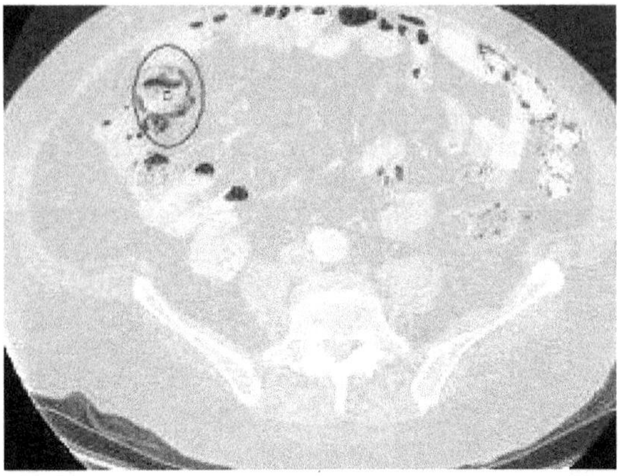

Figure 113. Axial CT of the pelvis in the same patient demonstrates bubbles of air in the wall of the small bowel called pneumatosis.

One extremely useful application is to identify intracranial hemorrhage or blood in the brain. This can be crucial to find, but AI also has false positives. For example, the AI called *Figure 114* an intracranial hemorrhage when it is a brain mass. The AI application looks for something bright to call a hemorrhage, so it highlighted the image below, even though it is actually a tumor.

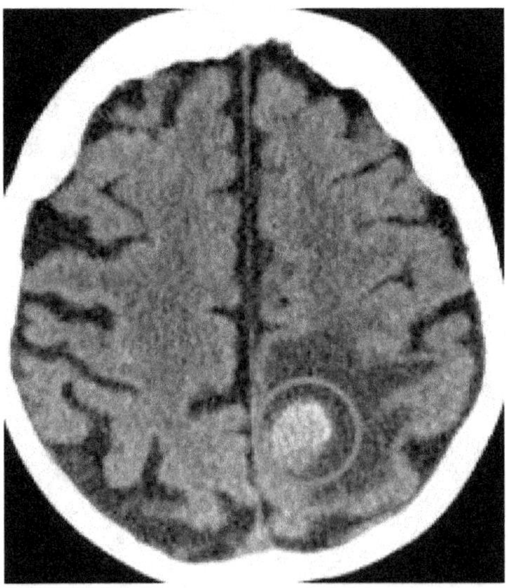

Figure 114. AI notifies that this image has a finding suspicious for an intracranial hemorrhage.

The surrounding dark grey is the vasogenic edema, associated with swelling of the brain cortex that is related to brain tumors. In this case the mass is likely a metastatic tumor. Below is what the tumor looks like on coronal images from the face to the back of the skull, contrasting to *Figure 114* on axial images from the top of the skull down to the neck.

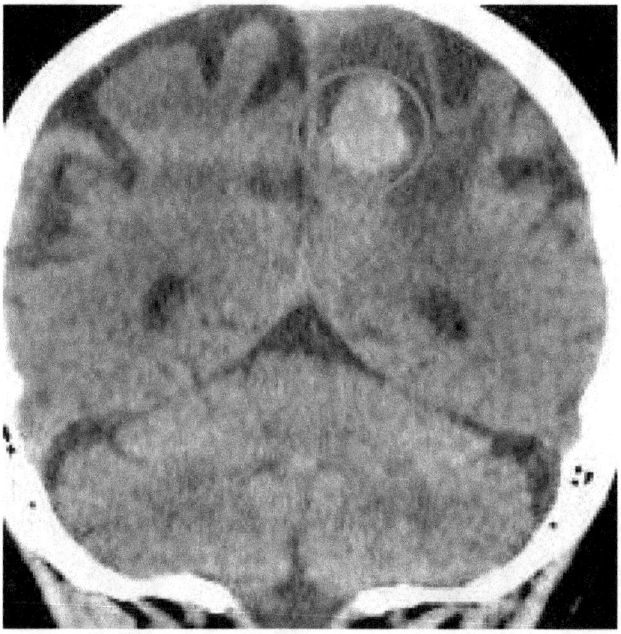

Figure 114. Coronal CT image of the brain demonstrating a left-brain mass (circled) with surrounding vasogenic edema (the grey around it). Notice that the grey does not extend to the surface of the brain, and this differentiates vasogenic edema associated with brain tumors from cytotoxic edema that is associated with brain infarcts.

In the next case (*Figure 115*) the AI does point out that there is suspicion for intracranial hemorrhage, but this is highlighting the bright line, circled, along the posterior aspect of the brain that is just related to the covering called the falx, a membrane that surrounds the skull. In this case, however, there is a hemorrhage, but it is in a different place to what is referenced.

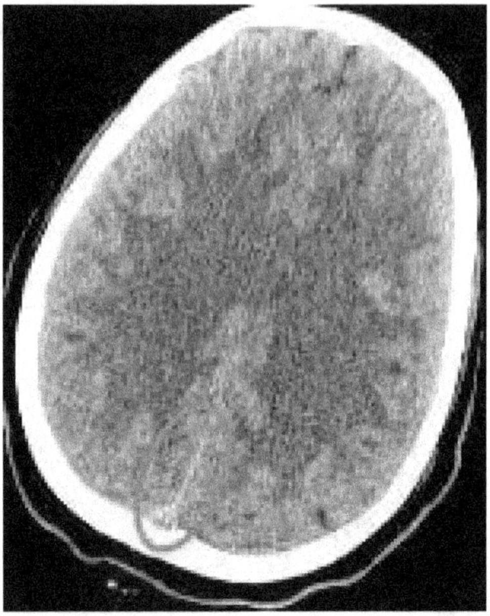

Figure 115. AI notifies that this image is suspicious for a brain hemorrhage (intracranial hemorrhage- ICH).

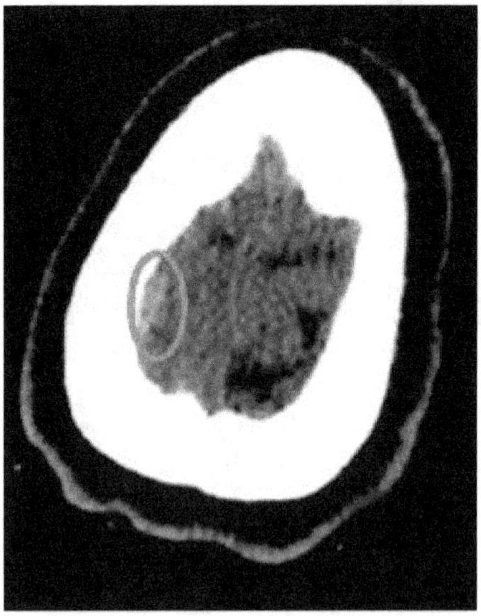

Figure 116. Axial CT of the right frontal lobe of the brain shows a small area of high density that represents a subtle small subdural hemorrhage. This is in a different area to the image that was the suspicious area reported by the AI application.

The real hemorrhage is called a subdural hemorrhage, which is high in the right frontal region, 3mm in width, and just beneath the scalp.

Below is the same subdural hemorrhage circled in the red in coronal view. Seeing the abnormalities on two different dimensional views can help confirm to the radiologist that the finding is real.

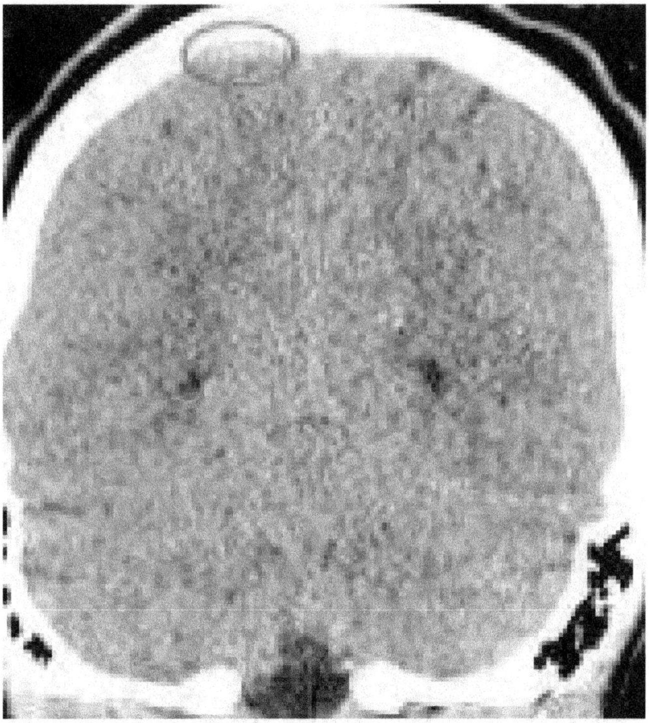

Figure 117. Coronal CT image with the tiny area of subdural hemorrhage circled at the top of the right brain.

In the following case (*Figure 118*), the AI correctly identified this intracranial (inside the brain) hemorrhage by pointing out the image, shown on the next page, for the radiologist to scrutinize. The hemorrhage in this case is inside the right lateral ventricle which is lit up. Since the hemorrhage does not have vasogenic edema or grey surrounding it, you can tell that this is not a tumor.

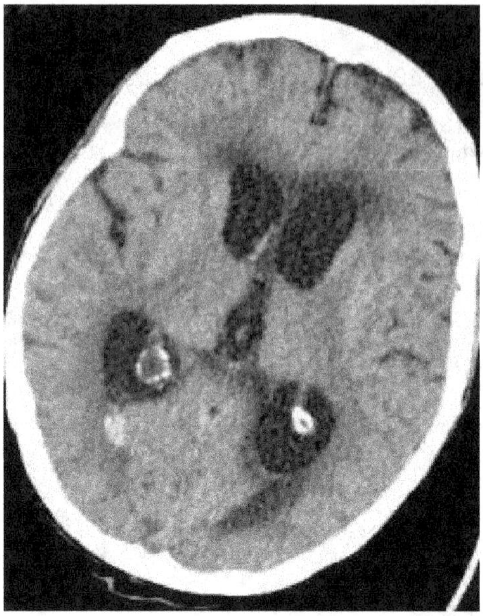

Figure 118. Axial CT notifies that this image has suspicion for intracranial hemorrhage.

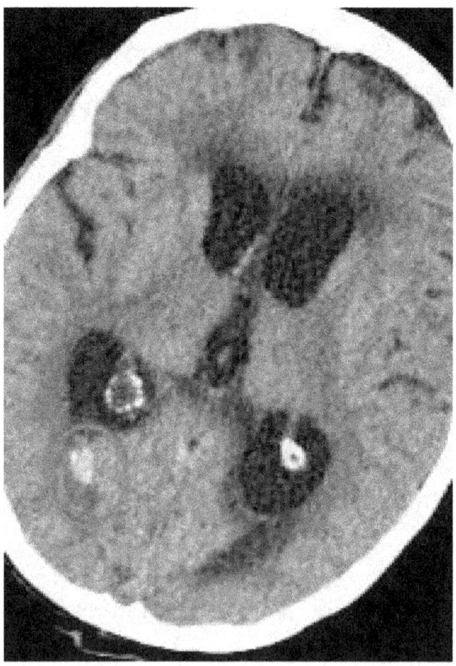

Figure 119. Circled is the area of intraventricular hemorrhage correctly identified by the AI application.

The AI called the example below an intracranial hemorrhage- but this large oval calcification is a meningioma along the midline. Additionally since it is as bright as the skull, it could not be a bleed, since bleeds are less dense.

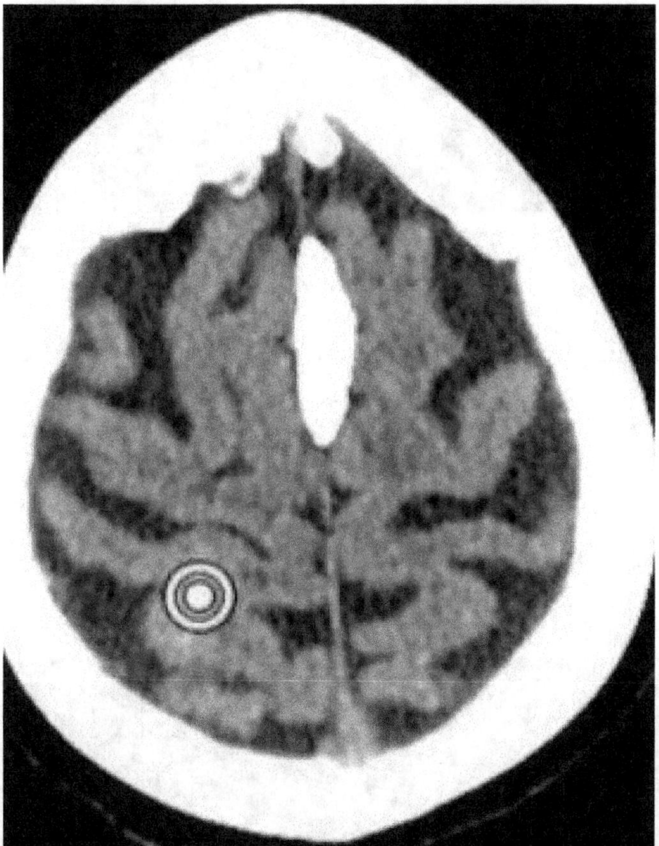

Figure 120. AI application notifies that this axial CT image is suspicious for containing intracranial hemorrhage, however this calcification along the midline is a calcified meningioma.

Another application that AI is used for is detecting subtle fractures. For example, *Figure 121* shows a subtle cervical spine fracture in C7 of the neck spine bones that the AI picked up.

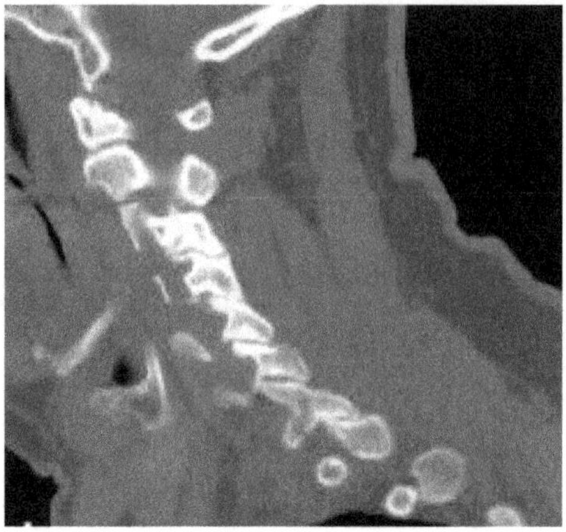

Figure 121. AI application notifies that this image is suspicious for a cervical spine fracture.

When examining this area closely, as seen in *Figure 122*, there was an additional C7 fracture - the more superior circled fracture was not detected by AI, but the AI was helpful in finding one of the fractures. The higher circle is showing the superior fracture, a larger vertical line, and the smaller circle beneath is displaying the fracture that the AI found.

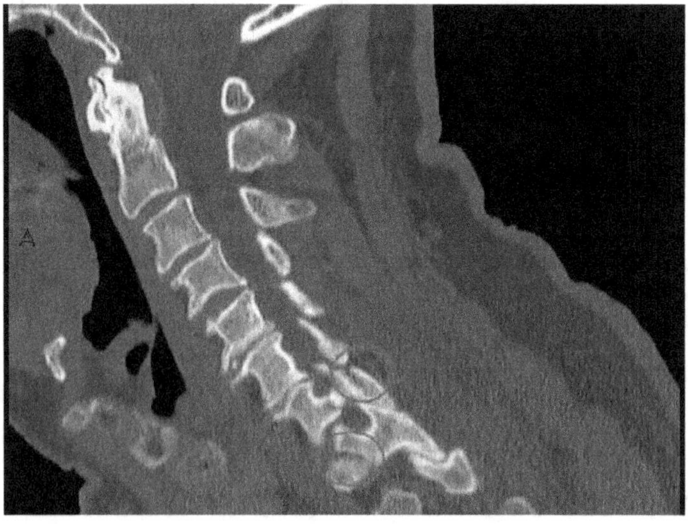

Figure 122. Two areas circled are fractures.

Another application that AI can be extremely useful for is in helping to find pulmonary nodules. These are spots in the lungs that are often benign and can be left alone. However, sometimes the nodules can grow, showing they could be malignant and represent lung cancer.

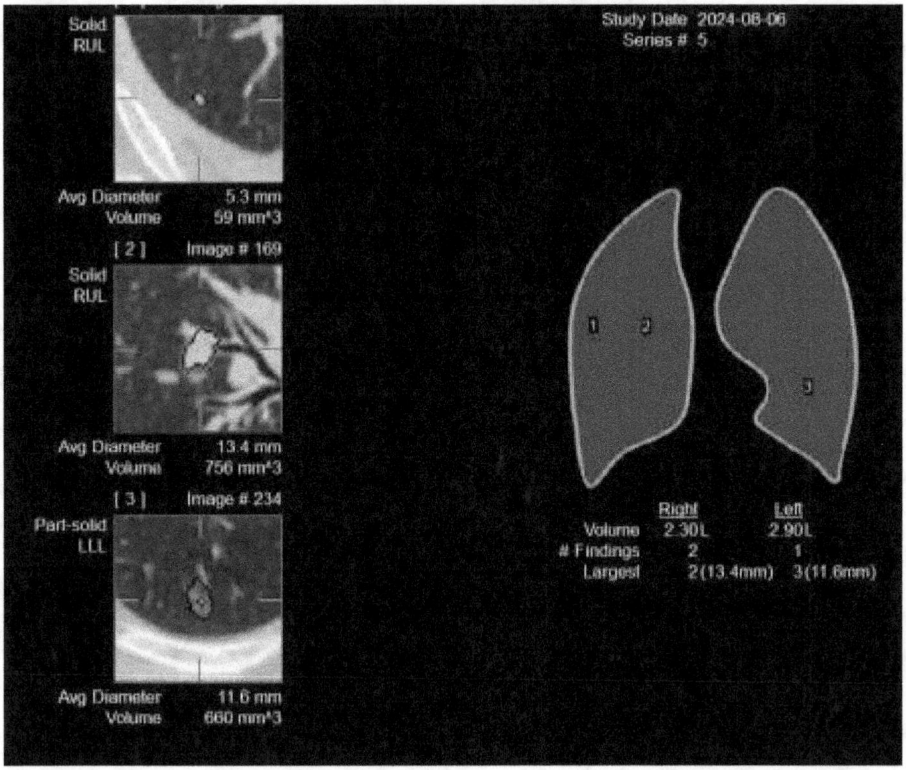

Figure 123. AI application depicts areas suspicious for pulmonary nodules.

This image directs the radiologist to look at all the areas the AI thinks there may be nodules. The larger one in the middle is shown in *Figure 124* on the original source CT.

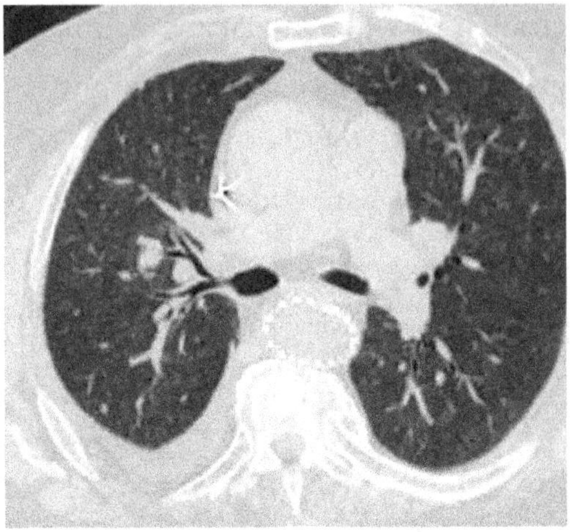

Figure 124. Circled is the largest of the pulmonary nodules detected by the AI application.

Now, one year ago when AI was not available for the application of finding pulmonary nodules, this area was not commented on by the radiologist in the prior report, but in retrospect there was a smaller and less dense (less white nodule) in this region, displayed in *Figure 125*. It has been growing since then and is now concerning for a small lung cancer. The patient already had another cancer resected a few years before and was on cancer surveillance, so you can see how AI can be a friend and not a threatening enemy by helping the radiologist.

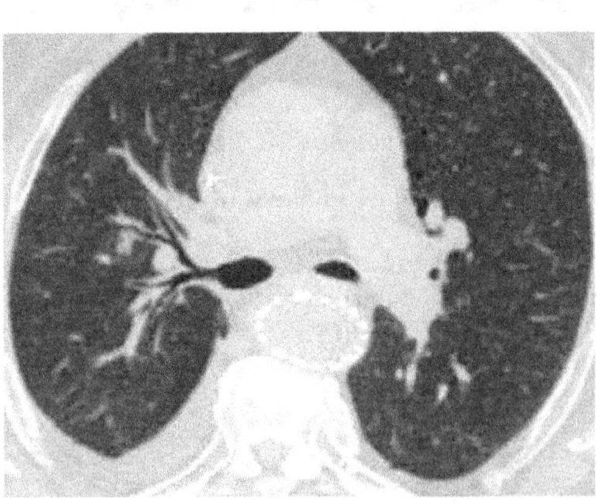

Figure 125. Axial CT image one year prior demonstrates a smaller size of the

nodule at that time where it was not picked up. Together with its growth this is suspicious for a small lung cancer.

Since the AI is not always precise, the radiologist is invaluable in making the correct diagnosis. The AI below called *Figure 126* a nodule. But when looking at the original source images on the CT scan, it can be seen to be the first rib junction.

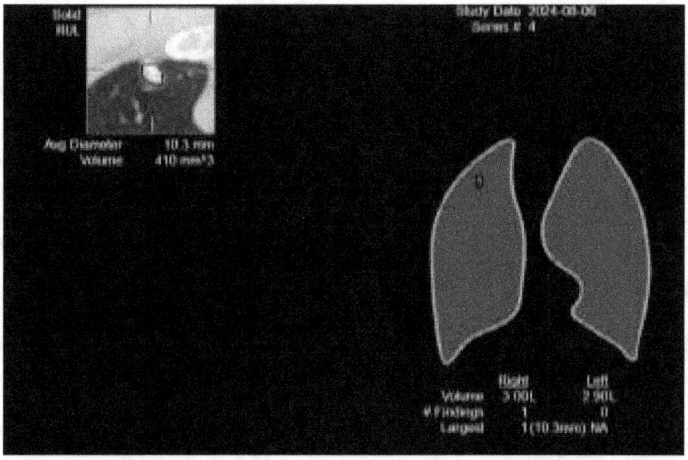

Figure 126. AI application reports suspicion for a nodule in the anterior right chest.

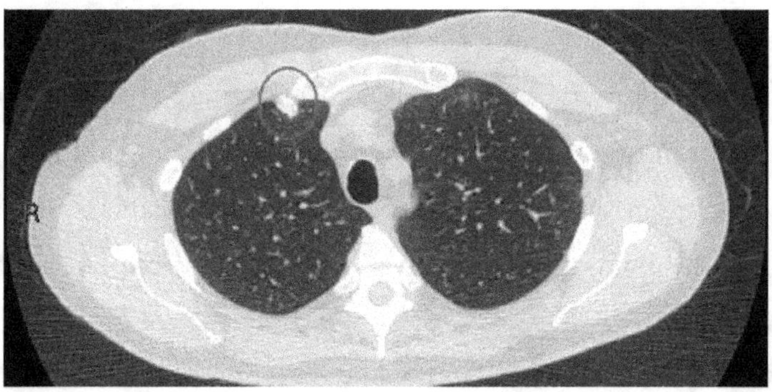

Figure 127. Scrutiny of this image demonstrates the suspicious area that is circled to represent the first costochondral junction- a common pitfall of the AI application.

You don't want the surgeon to take out your first rib just because the computer said that it was a nodule. That would not be cool!

CHAPTER 8

WHAT IS A RADIOLOGIST? MYTHS DEBUNKED

WHAT ARE SOME MYTHS ABOUT RADIOLOGY?

RADIOLOGISTS STAY IN A DARK ROOM ALL DAY

Don't worry—radiologists are nothing like Darth Vader, who constantly wears a mask and is notoriously anti-social. Although a radiologist does work in a dimly lit room, the reading room is a fun and jovial environment, where radiologists interact and socialize in their break time or in between analyzing studies. They can do this with fellow radiologists and other members of the healthcare team. In addition, many hospitals have trainees, so teaching is also a role one can perform in the hospital.

RADIOLOGISTS NEVER SEE OR TALK TO PATIENTS

There are some sub-specialties where the radiologist must talk to patients to perform their procedures or inform them about the next step in imaging or biopsies. The radiologist can choose to have a more interactive type of sub-specialty if they desire. The best part, however, is that the radiologist only must deal with the imaging procedure at hand, and the rest of the patient's problems—i.e., all the aches and pains—are managed by their primary doctor, who would have ordered the procedure. The radiologist acts as the doctor's doctor. Clinical teams often drop into radiology as part of their rounds, to figure out what is going on with their patient. The emergency doctor is dependent on the radiologist to determine whether a patient is free to be released home or needs to be admitted to the hospital.

RADIOLOGY IS BORING

Radiology is the most dynamic specialty in medicine, taking advantage of many new innovations and advances. There is and always has been continued growth in the field, which is tied to the growth of the computer industry. It is not just about reading boring X-rays. With the current degree of precision and high-resolution images now able to be obtained, the day's work is filled with beautiful images and the excitement of solving puzzles, making diagnoses that are critical to the patient's health. If you enjoy being a detective or solving problems, radiology may be a perfect fit.

RADIOLOGISTS ARE ANTI-SOCIAL INTROVERTS WHO ARE AFRAID OF TALKING TO PEOPLE

Depending on the person, radiologists can be fun, social, and extroverted. Communication lies at the heart of radiology, as practitioners are in constant communication with the ordering/primary doctors, whether it be via emails or phone calls or in person to review images. Radiologists' favorite time is socializing amongst themselves, as they often share a similar type of personality. So, if you find that radiology appeals to you, it is very likely you will find friends in the reading room.

THE RADIOLOGY JOB MARKET IS BAD, AND GETTING A JOB IS DIFFICULT. IN A FEW YEARS, ARTIFICIAL INTELLIGENCE IS GOING TO TAKE OVER RADIOLOGY AND YOUR ROLE

There is a global shortage of radiologists, which has been the case for a long time. Radiologists receive numerous offers for permanent roles or temporary jobs (locums). There is also huge flexibility because of the significant demand. So many radiologists can choose to work from home some or all of the time, using reading stations connected to high-speed internet, if they desire. This makes it a perfect career for people with caring responsibilities, such as those with young children or elderly relatives. Hours are becoming increasingly flexible.

Additionally, artificial intelligence (AI) is not an evil villain who is waiting to take away the radiologist's job. In fact, radiologists have an enthusiasm for AI, as its developing capabilities aids their efficiency. It is a helpful tool that can help to confirm a radiologist's suspicion, point the radiologist in a certain direction; or highlight subtle abnormalities. However, it cannot replace a human that has spent many years in training to perform this job. In addition, AI cannot perform biopsies, drainages, and injections. Radiologists are here to stay.

RADIOLOGISTS ARE CONSISTENTLY EXPOSED TO HAZARDOUS LEVELS OF RADIATION

Only a few of the sub-specialties such as interventional radiology require the radiologist to be anywhere close to radiation. Tools are in effect to minimize radiation exposure and the safety of the radiologist. Instead of a cooking apron to protect against messy spills, the radiologist wears a lead apron to stop the X-rays from going into their body. Many of the imaging tests do not even use radiation such as ultrasound and MRI. Most of the radiologists are working in front of a bunch of computers like playing a video game all day long and are not exposed to radiation.

RADIOLOGISTS ARE MOSTLY WOMEN.

Radiology has been underrepresented by women over several decades being relatively consistent at around a quarter of the United States radiology residents being women. This is a stark difference when compared to specialties such as family medicine, pediatrics, geriatrics, obstetrics/gynecology, dermatology, and psychiatry where women represent a sizable portion or even dominate certain areas. Leadership roles for women in radiology are even lower with fewer than 10% of department chairs being women. Women have represented a large portion of medical students for multiple years and now compromise the majority- making up 54.6% of all medical students in the United States from 2023 to 2024, yet this does not translate into the number of women entering radiology residency. So what are the reasons for this disparity? Medical students have reported in surveys the perceived lack of patient contact as a reason why women did not pursue radiology. However, this cannot be the entire explanation as the specialty of pathology, which constitutes even less patient contact than radiology, has a higher percentage of women physicians. Other factors cited include the competitiveness of the specialty and its requirements of physics knowledge. In addition, radiation exposure, lack of acknowledgement by patients, working in a dark room and little if any prior insight into the daily practices of the field have been cited as factors in the gender disparity for radiology. Hopefully, this book may open the eyes of both women and men to understand that intellectual stimulation, a conducing work environment and impact on patient care are important benefits of radiology, factors that have shown to contribute to the attraction of radiology for many students.

RADIOLOGY IS EASY

Every doctor thinks they can read an X-ray, but radiology is much more than that. MRI interpretation needs specialized training, and CT scans can be a lot more complicated than the surgeon may expect. What the surgeon may believe to be the stomach may be the colon in actuality! How chaotic would it be if the surgeon removed the wrong organ? As mentioned previously, the radiologist is the doctor's doctor. They are knowledgeable in the diagnosis and treatment of all varieties of patient (from infants to elderly) and get to be involved in all of the interesting cases of the hospital. There is a reason why the field of radiology is so competitive, and why only hardworking, studious, and dedicated medical students can get into this residency. It's a long road to becoming a radiologist, with undergraduate education and then medical school needed, followed by residency and then possibly a year of fellowship. However, the rewards are huge, both in terms of the satisfaction of solving mysteries and the financial return. Radiologists typically make higher salaries than other medical professionals. Overall, it's a dream job, but one must be prepared to work hard to reach the gold.

CONCLUSION

Radiology is a fascinating, challenging and continuously changing career- a career option that many people including those entering medical school have little insight into or awareness of. This book is aimed at shedding light upon a career not often considered. When one thinks of becoming a doctor or what the typical life of a doctor is like, one is not often considering the career of a radiologist. It is a hidden gem. One must have a passion for their career, and it would be best for them to feel like they are doing something they love to do every day. Most radiologists are happy with their career, and many are still working even after age 80 despite the lack of need for money, which exemplifies the rewarding nature of this speciality. The new innovations and constantly evolving technology make it a career that never sleeps but continues to be challenging and continues to engage the brain.

Some of the benefits of becoming a radiologist are a flexible schedule, an excellent work life balance, as well as opportunities for advancement and for teaching (for example in a teaching program to train residents). Despite the rumors of Artificial intelligence taking over the field of radiology, there is no fear of that in the radiology world and overall, the future is positive. Fascinating duties make up the typical workday with freedom from a boring routine. Everyday a radiologist is helping others, making life altering decisions and an impact on hundreds of people's lives, so they receive huge satisfaction. The job is secure and stable. With huge flexibility, the radiologist can also choose in which setting they would prefer to work, whether it be at home, hybrid, at a hospital, or doing procedures all day long. Since there is a large shortage with the future boding continued shortages in the radiologist's workforce, there are a wide variety of options for off hours shifts which can bring in extra days off where radiologist can relax or make even more money working if they desire.

The disadvantages of becoming a radiologist include lengthy education and training, large workload especially in busy healthcare settings, high stress and pressure- one is making critical, and life changing diagnoses based on images of the patient. The accuracy of the interpretation can have a serious impact on patient care and sometimes for radiologists can lead to burn out. A sedentary work environment can be viewed as a disadvantage but also can be seen as an advantage for choosing lifestyle and flexibility. Compared to other medical specialties, radiologists have limited direct patient contact with much of the work involving interpreting images and collaborating with other physicians and co-workers. Again, this can be seen as a positive.

When considering career options, radiology is often an unfamiliar and uncontemplated career. Probing more into this career may offer opportunities one may have not ever thought about. This book is just a glance/glimpse into CT's used in radiology, but so many more modalities of imaging are available as part of the job including ultrasound, MRI, plain X-rays, fluoroscopy, interventional procedures, and nuclear medicine. Remember, no job is boring if you love what you do and that is what you should be in search of when thinking about what the best career path for you is.

ABOUT THE AUTHOR

Sophia Aishwarya Li, born and brought up in Los Angeles California is a 15-year-old whose life changed during a summer whilst volunteering at a nearby hospital. She is hoping to open your eyes to the possibility of a life changing career that she is motivated to pursue herself. Whilst wandering through the radiology reading room on her way to delivering gifts from the gift shop, she happened to discover that one could see inside humans-their anatomy, what was normal and what was abnormal –crisp and clear as if it were on a television screen, all without surgery, without blood, grease, or dirt but in the luxury of a beautiful though dim lit reading room. She was hooked! The intrigue blossomed to her pursuit of educating more people about this hidden gem of a career especially students like herself, talented and motivated, trying to find a career path that could lead to happiness in their adult life. Subsequently she went to work, learning more about radiology including obtaining images from teaching files from helpful residents, and advice from renowned radiologists. YouTube videos that Sophia has created have been featured on the UCanbehealthierTV channel to inspire young adults with career aspirations to consider this high demand, rewarding though challenging career that has rewards greater than money or lifestyle alone. This book aims to share, with any child or aspiring medical student, the passion she has in discovering the endless beauties of radiology– a little-known or thought of career when considering becoming a doctor.

www.ingramcontent.com/pod-product-compliance
Lightning Source LLC
LaVergne TN
LVHW022229200926
848481LV00006B/2182
* 9 7 9 8 3 4 8 5 8 5 1 1 2 *